Musculos
Examination.

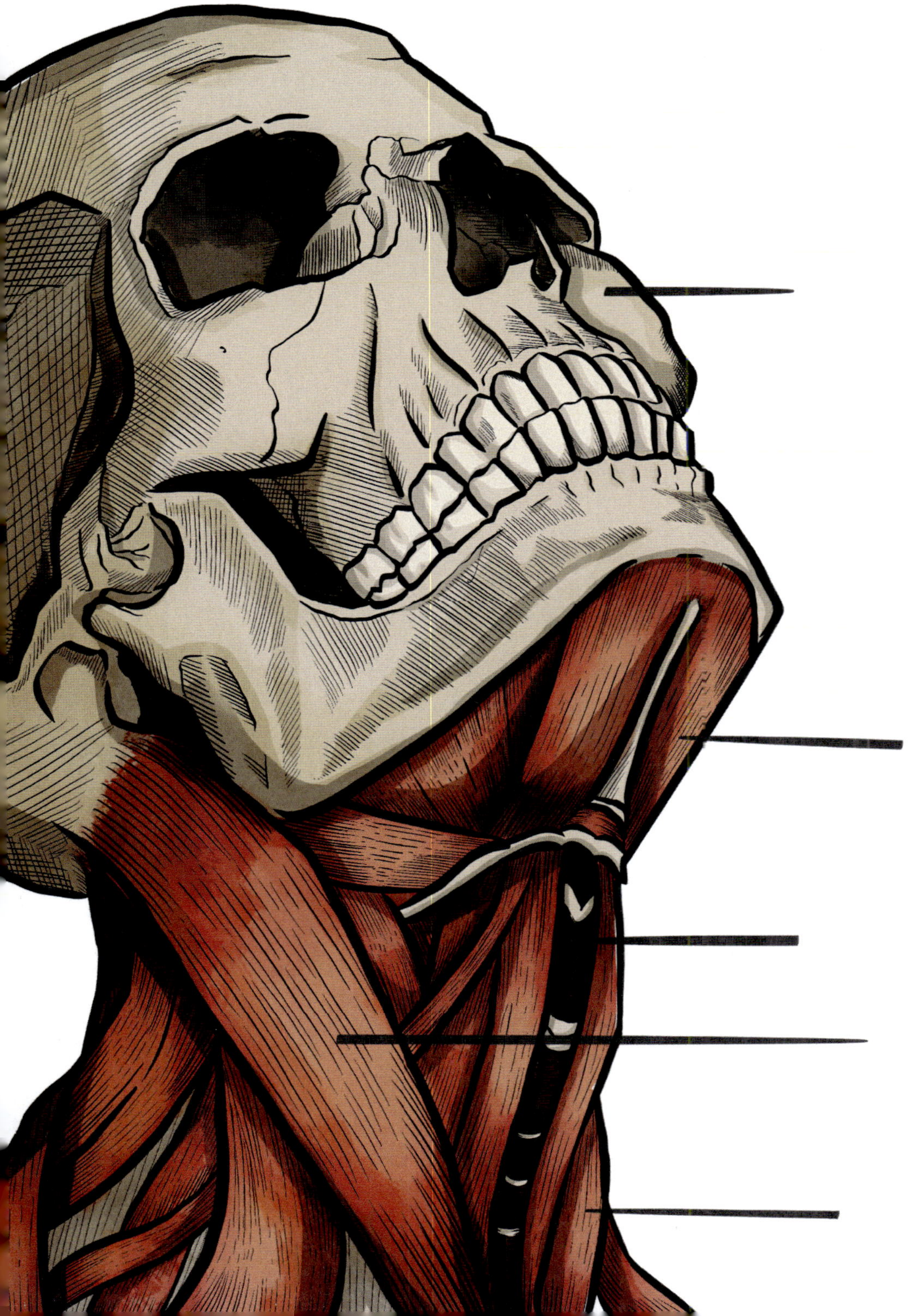

OSCE Unlocked.

Dr Katriona Hutchison - Dr Barrie Lyell - Dr Riya Thomas - Dr Laura Brown - Dr Jack Wellington - Dr Michael Carvill

Dedication

This book is dedicated to all of our friends and family who spent hours helping us revise for our OSCEs. We hope this guide will assist current and future medical students in developing their examination skills.

We would also like to thank the Graphics team at Medic Mentor for their incredible creativity and vision in illustrating this book and helping make it a reality.

This edition published in 2023 by Mentor Publishing

A catalogue record for this book is available from the British Library

Written by Dr Katriona Hutchison - Dr Barrie Lyell - Dr Riya Thomas - Dr Laura Brown - Dr Jack Wellington - Dr Michael Carvill

Illustrations by Bex Sutton - Tembalbazali Ncube - Lorna Davey - Michael Rogers

ISBN
Paperback: 978-1-7384566-0-4
Ebook: 978-1-7384566-1-1

OSCE Unlocked.

Contents

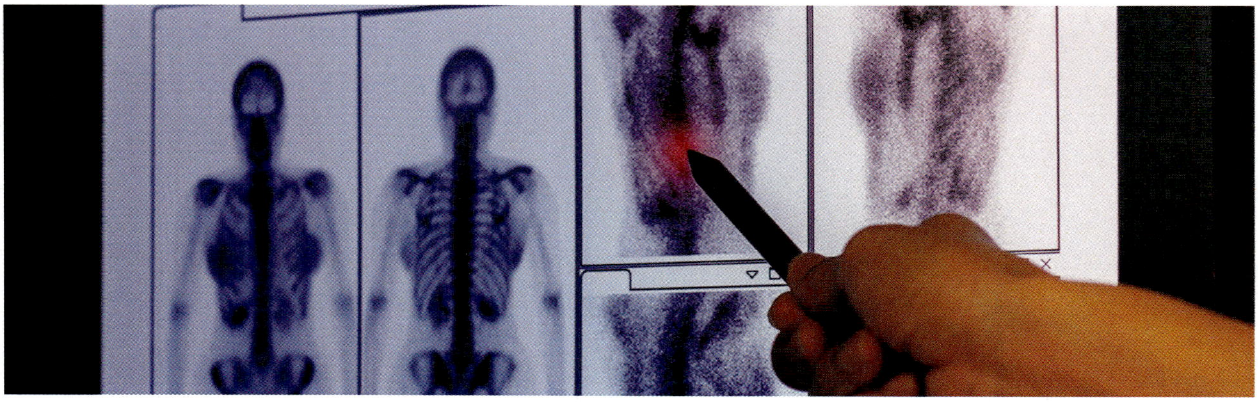

Chapter 1: Introduction

Dr Laura Brown MbChB

Muscles are essential to every aspect of human life, whilst bones provide protection, structure and shape to the human body. The main functions of the musculoskeletal system are stability, protection, support, and movement. However, the musculoskeletal system is more complex than often initially appreciated and in addition to its core functions it also has an essential role in blood cell production, mineral storage, heat production, glycogen storage and maintaining posture.

The musculoskeletal system can be divided into two parts: muscular and skeletal, or more simply the muscles and bones.

There are approximately 600 muscles in the body which can be subdivided into 3 subtypes: smooth, skeletal and cardiac. For the purposes of this book we will focus on skeletal muscles. Skeletal muscles are considered the main functional component of the muscular system. Skeletal muscles are defined by the following characteristics: excitability, contractility, extensibility and elasticity. It is these muscles that work in tandem the neurological system to provide the body with the ability to move.

The skeletal system is primarily made up of bone. When two (or more) bones meet, they form a joint. Together with the ligaments and tendons this forms a skeletal structure that is not only strong enough to provide protection but also allows delicate mobilisation.

Aside from the bones and muscles the musculoskeletal system also consists of cartilage, tendons, ligaments and connective tissue. A tendon is a tough fibrous tissue that attaches bone to muscle allowing transmission of mechanical forces and thus producing limb movements. Ligaments, in contrast, connect bone to bone often providing stability to joints. Cartilage is avascular, firm, yet softer than bone, and functions as “shock absorber” throughout the musculoskeletal system. Lastly, connective tissue is an umbrella term that includes a variety of different tissues that hold, separate, bind, connect, protect and give a supportive framework to joints.

Joints

Joints can be classified based on the type of connective tissue present (fibrous, cartilaginous, or synovial), or by the degree of movement at the joint (synarthrosis, amphiarthrosis, and diathrosis). Fibrous joints allow minimal to no movement as they are constrained by dense fibrous tissue. Cartilaginous joints vary from allowing no movement to some movement depending on the type of cartilage present in the joint. Synovial joints allow a wide range of movement within specific planes, these joints are the foundation of the musculoskeletal system.

There are a multitude of synovial joints which can be subdivided into the types based on the movements they allow. The direction and extent of movement is determined by the articular surfaces of the joint in addition to the muscle and ligaments which act to stabilise and limit movement in alternative planes.

Types of Synovial Joints:

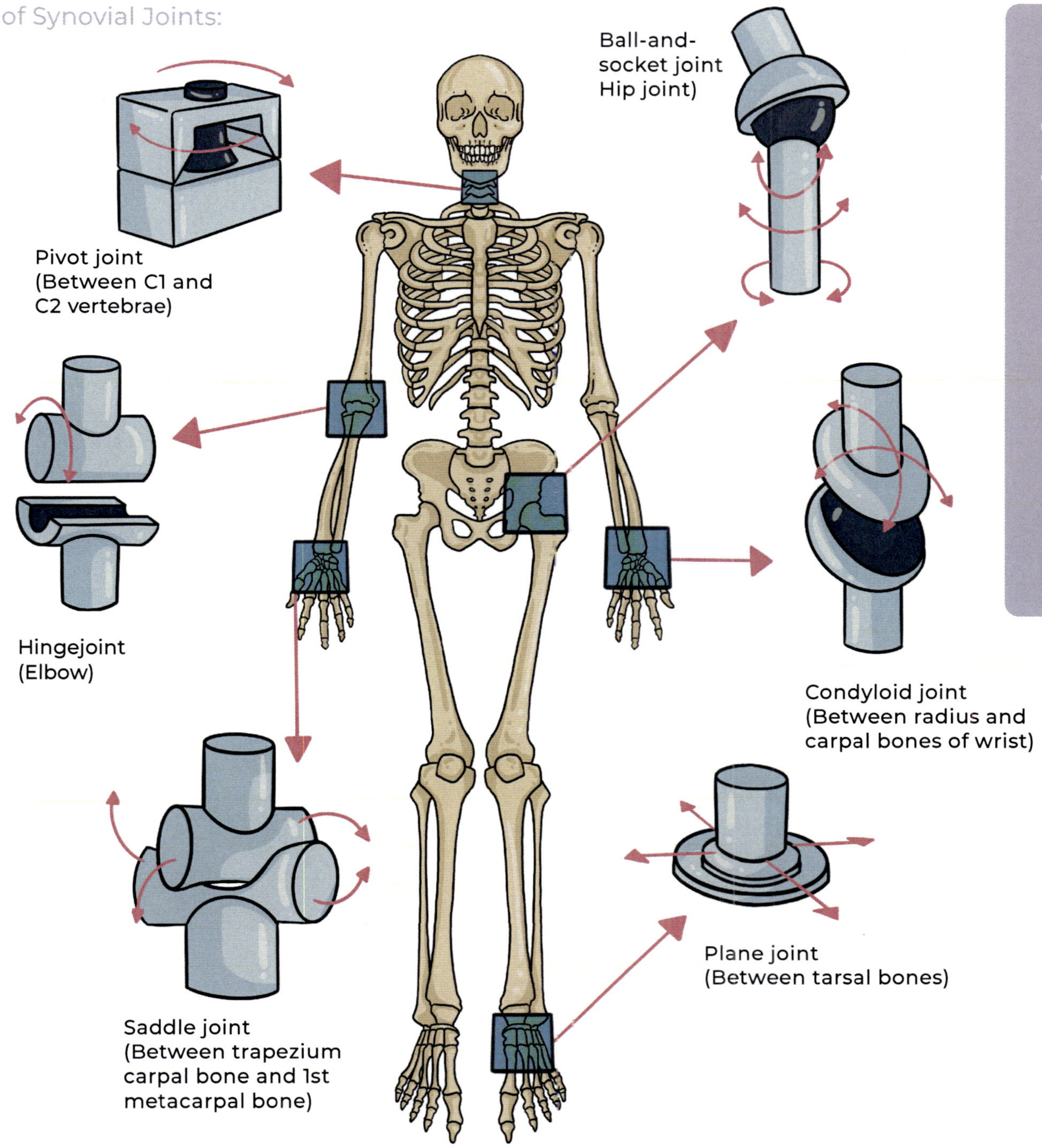

Joint Classification	Possible Movements	Example
Hinge	Flexion, Extension	Elbow, Ankle
Saddle	Flexion, Extension, Abduction, Adduction and Circumduction	1st Carpometacarpal Joint
Plane	Sliding/Gliding Movements	Subtalar Joint, Vertebral Facet Joints
Ball and Socket	Flexion, Extension, Abduction, Adduction, External Rotation, and Internal Rotation	Shoulder, Hip
Pivot	Rotation	Atlantoaxial Joint, Proximal and Distal Radioulnar Joints
Condyloid (ellipsoid)	Flexion, Extension, Abduction, Adduction and Circumduction	Metacarpophalangeal Joints, Radiocarpal joints

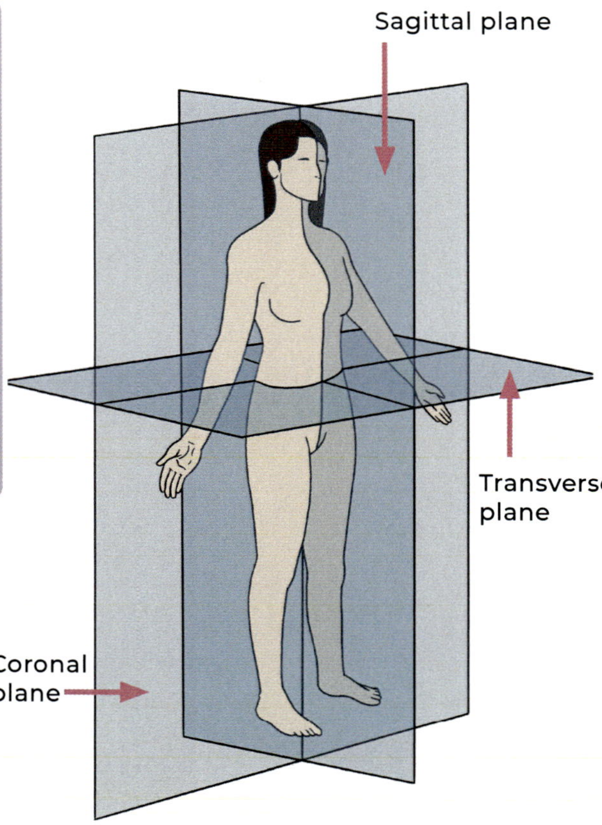

When describing movements of joints or limbs it is important that one always starts with the anatomical position.

The anatomical position describes the following stance: standing upright vertically with head and eyes directed straight forwards, upper limbs are held slightly away from the trunk with palms facing forwards, thumbs are pointing away from the trunk, lower limbs are parallel with feet firmly flat on the ground with feet and toes facing forwards.

Only from this position can planes of movement be consistently described and understood. The three most common planes include sagittal, coronal and transverse. To understand and visualise the sagittal plane, picture the human body in the anatomical position, then draw and imaginary, vertical line down the midline of the body dividing the body into left and right sides. The coronal plane is another vertical plane that is perpendicular and (90 degrees) to the sagittal plane. For the coronal plane, begin again with the body in the anatomical position and then draw an imaginary line through the middle of the head intersecting the ears and down through the body, dividing the body into front and back (anterior and posterior). Finally, the transverse plane or axial plane is horizontal and parallel to the ground. Imagine drawing an imaginary horizantal line across the torso, dividing the body into the top and bottom, or upper and lower sections.

Description of movements always start in the anatomical position. Most movements have an opposite movement and these opposing pairs can be grouped together.

Flexion and Extension

- These movements occur within the sagittal plane.
- Flexion reduces the angle between two body parts and extension increases it.
- For example, from the anatomical position, moving the hand towards the shoulder will result in elbow flexion. Knee flexion occurs in contrast when moving the heel of the foot from the anatomical position towards the buttock.

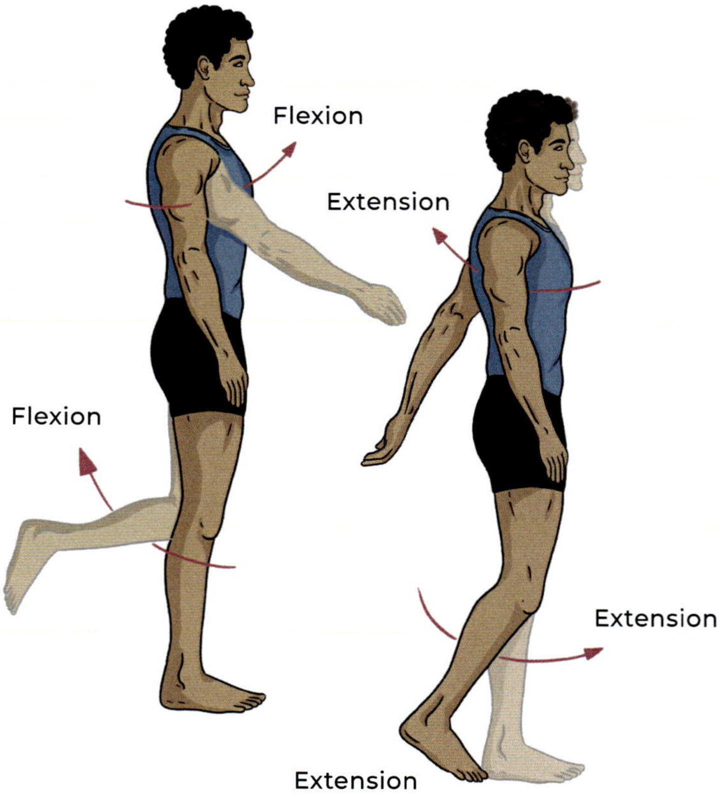

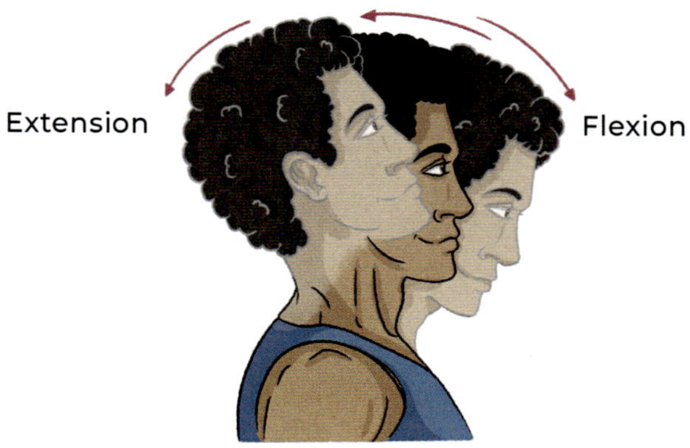

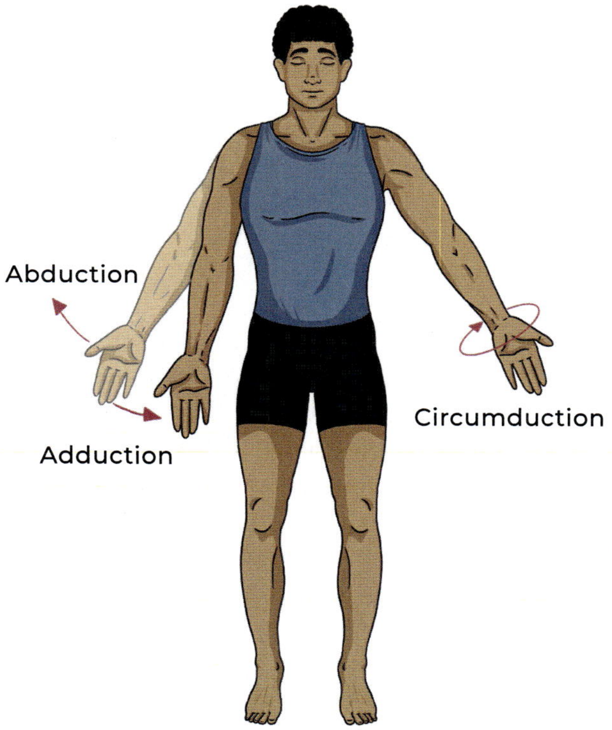

Abduction and Adduction:

- These motions take place in the coronal plane of movement. Abduction describes movement away from the midline, whilst adduction describes movement towards the midline.
- For example, moving the arm away laterally from the body is abduction, whilst moving the arm towards the midline is adduction.

Medial (internal) and Lateral (external) Rotation:

- Internal rotation involves rotation of a limb inwardly towards the midline and lateral rotation involves rotation outwardly away from the midline.

For example, the image below depicts Internal and External Rotation of the hip:

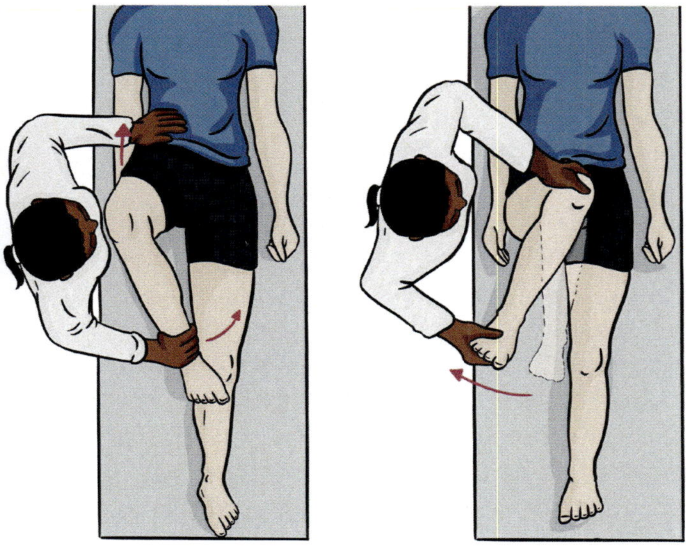

Pronation and Supination:

When a person lies flat, on their back, this called the supine position. If one turnws over to lay face down this can be described as being in the prone position.

These movements also describe the movement of the forearm. Supination describes the elbow being flexed to 90 degrees and turning the hand so the palm is facing upwards. Pronation describes a flexed elbow with the palm facing downwards.

Circumduction:

Describes a circular movement of a joint, that involves flexion, extension ,abduction and adduction. This is seen at the 1st carpometacarpal joint.

Opposition and Reposition:

Opposition describes the ability to move the thumb to touch the distal aspect of a finger. Reposition is the opposing movement: the thumb returning back to its usual anatomical position.

Inversion and Eversion:

These movements that occur at the ankle joint. Inversion is when the sole of the foot points towards the midline and eversion is when the sole of the foot points away from the midline.

Dorsiflexion and Plantar flexion:

The dorsum of the foot refers to the top/superior aspect of the foot and the plantar surface is the inferior/sole of the foot.

Dorsiflexion is aptly named as it is flexion towards the dorsal surface; likewise, plantarflexion is flexion towards the plantar surface.

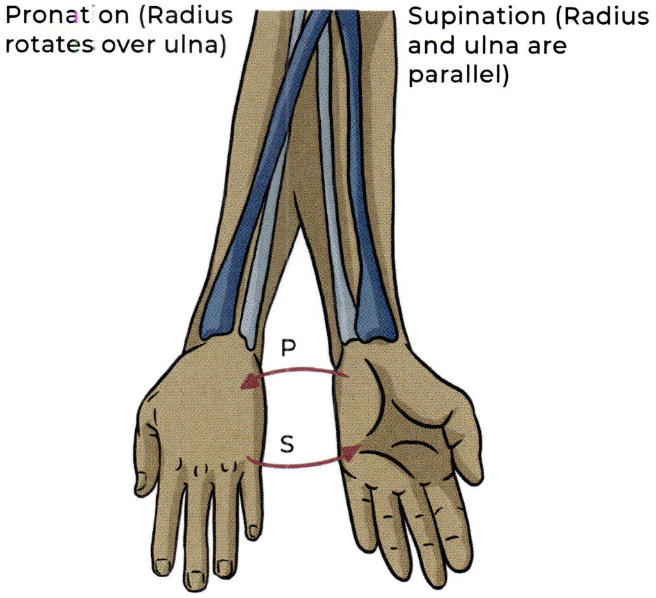

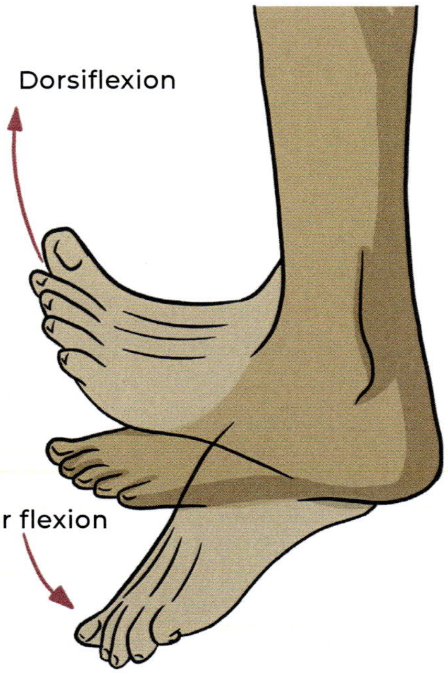

Principles of Joint Examination

Effective assessment of joints is crucial in identifying pathology and correctly diagnosing and managing patients with musculoskeletal presenting complaints. A simple structure of Look, Feel and Move can form the basis of all joint examinations in non-urgent clinical medicine; major trauma is not discussed within this book.

This book will focus on common musculoskeletal pathology; however, a physician should always consider and exclude life threatening pathology at first instance. There are many medical conditions that can mimic musculoskeletal problems such as, jaw/chest/shoulder pain from a myocardial infarction, shoulder pain secondary to a gastrointestinal perforation, back pain from an aortic dissection or limb weakness due to stroke. Furthermore, major joint dislocations with neurovascular compromise, suspected septic joints, compartment syndrome and cauda equina all require immediate emergency medical attention, and are beyond the scope of this book.

A detailed and full history is required prior to examination. After initial assessment, if the patient is in a stable condition, the look, feel, move approach can help to provide a basis for a thorough musculoskeletal examination.

Look:

It is important to remember that the examination of the musculoskeletal system begins long before a patient is touched. The examination starts by simply observing the patient. This is best done by observing the patient generally and then focussing on the specific and relevant area of the body.

General:

Pay attention to how the patient mobilises from the waiting room. How did the patient arrive at the department or clinic? If the patient is known to the physician, do they seem far from their baseline? Do they appear in pain? Are there any obvious asymmetries? How does the patient sit down and mobilise? What is the patient's posture like? Are they using any walking aids? Are there any bandages or support dressings in situ? An excellent physician would have observed the patient thoroughly before the patient had sat down in the consultation room.

Specific:

Expose the area to be examined, always including the joints above and below the area in question as often pathologies can be referred from surrounding joints. Inspect the areas for any scars, swellings, injuries, deformities, erythema or discolouration.

Feel:

Prior to palpation always ask the patient if they have any pain. Palpation should begin by assessing the joint with the back of the hand to detect changes in temperature between the joint itself and its surrounding areas.

The neurovascular status of the limb should be assessed through palpation of the pulses, assessment of capillary refill and examination of sensation throughout all relevant dermatomes.

Subsequently, palpation of the joint and its surrounding areas, using the palmar aspect of the physician's hand is utilised to find swellings, any irregular tissue or bony abnormalities. Fine details of the bony landmarks and joint surfaces should then be examined using fingertips to palpate for any deformities of the joint and its surroundings. Knowing the 'normal' anatomy of the joint is paramount to identifying abnormalities.

Take note of when tenderness is elicited, by observing the patient's facial expressions throughout the examination. This is essential as patients do not always verbalise when they are in discomfort.

Move:

The range of movement of the joint is assessed actively (the patient moving their own limb) and passively (with the physician mobilising the joint independently from the patient).

Any pain, reduction in range of movement or weakness should be noted.

Special Tests:

Special tests for certain joints should be employed when relevant to elicit joint-specific signs and their relevant pathologies.

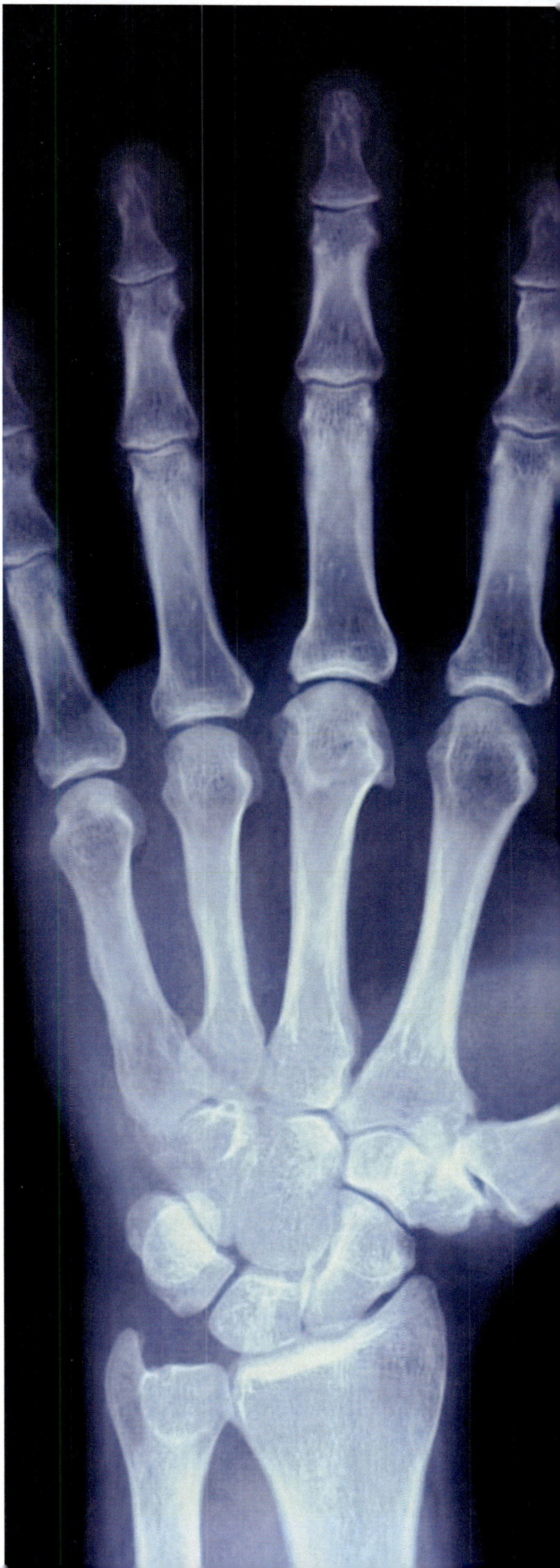

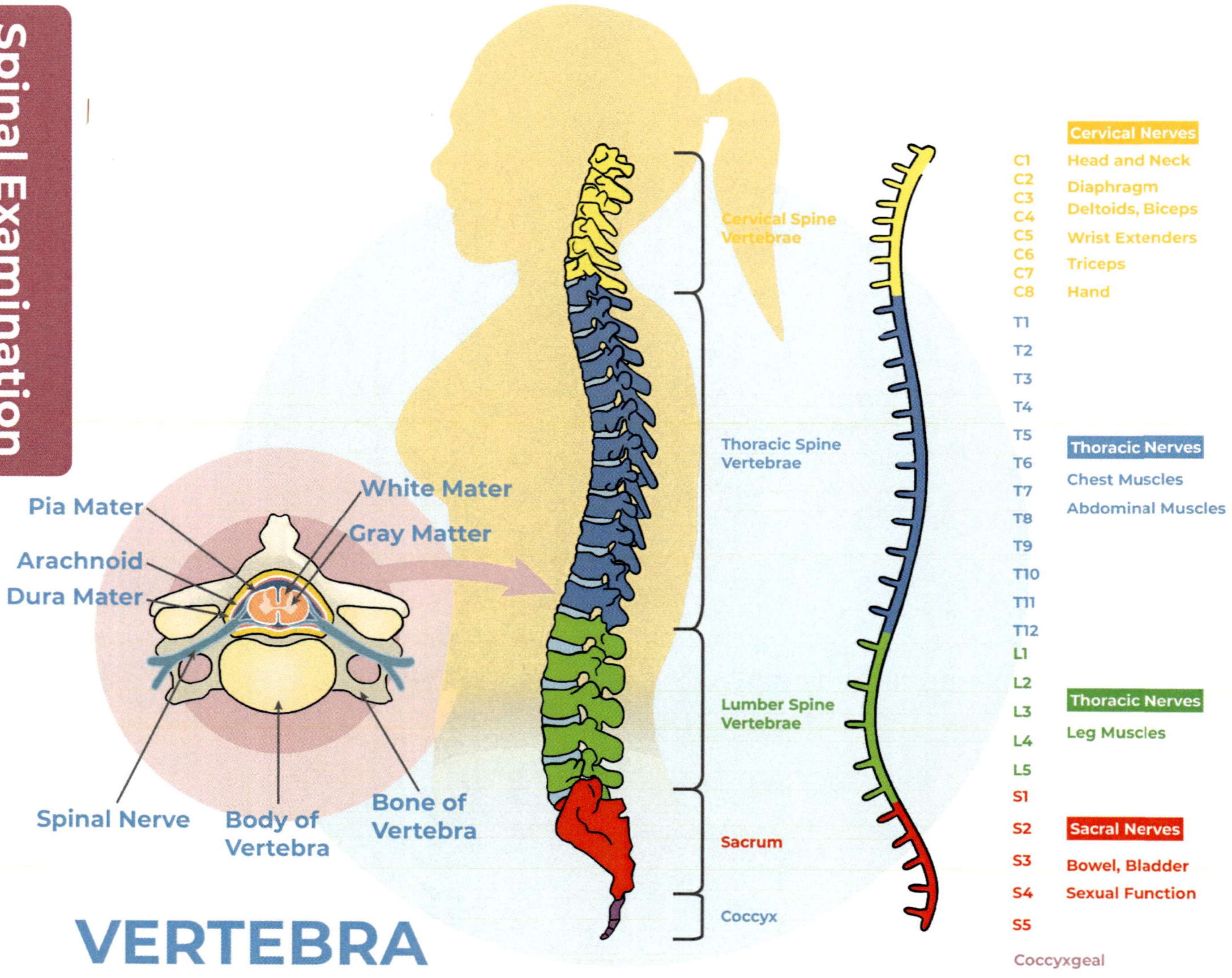

Chapter 2: Spinal Examination

Dr Jack Wellington MBBCh (Hons) MSc (LSHTM) FGMS FRSA

The spine, or vertebral column, is what determines animal diversity, dividing vertebrates from invertebrates. The spine is central component of the axial skeleton of vertebrates. Its primary function is to provide protection to the spinal cord of the central nervous system. In addition, the spinal column facilitates truncal movement through the various divisions of the spine, i.e., the cervical, thoracic, lumbar, and sacral spine. The spine is composed of vertebrae separated by fibrocartilaginous intervertebral discs which cushion the spinal joints and facets. This structure, provides rigidity and stability for the body's weight against gravitational and external forces.

Although an essential component of the axial skeleton, the spine is inflicted by a plethora of pathologies, most commonly musculoskeletal in origin. Such conditions involve osteoarthritic and traumatic processes (i.e., degenerative cervical myelopathy, cauda equina syndrome), autoimmune aetiologies (i.e., ankylosing spondylitis), infection (i.e., discitis), and neoplastic transformation (i.e., multiple myeloma and bony metastases).

When examining the spine, the following guide can be used to ensure a detailed and effective assessment of the patient.

As with all examinations – start by washing your hands, introducing yourself to the patient, checking the patient details, explanation of the examination and gaining consent. Subsequently ask the patient to expose the upper body and stand whilst maintaining patient dignity.

LOOK

General Inspection

Patient

- Do they appear unwell, uncomfortable, in pain/discomfort?
- Are there any obvious spinal deformities?
- Are there any signs of trauma?
- Assess general age, body habitus, and any obvious muscle atrophy.

Patient's Surroundings

- Are there any mobility aids or a spinal brace in the patient's vicinity?
- Assess the patient's footwear.

Inspection of Gait

Gait should be assessed when the patient enters the room (if mobilising)

- Is the patient using walking aids?
  - Assess the speed the patient is walking at, the stride length and for any obvious leg length discrepancies.
- Inspect the phases of the gait cycle:
  - Heel-strike → Foot flat → Mid-stance → Heel-off→ Toe-off→ Swing
- Look for abnormalities when turning.
- Look for any gait abnormalities.
  - Trendelenburg's Gait - superior gluteal nerve lesion / L5 radiculopathy (see image below)

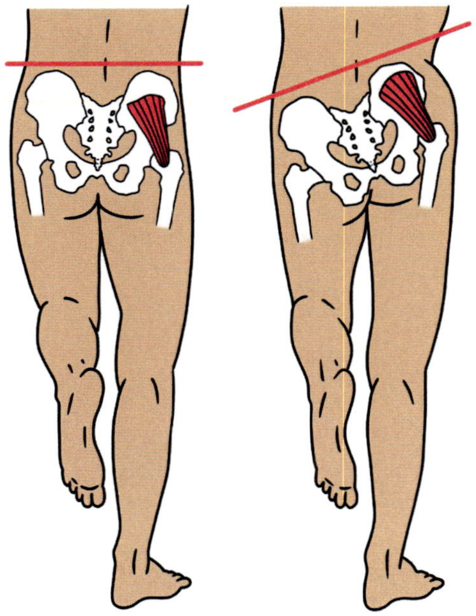

Trendelenburg's Gait

  - Waddling Gait - bilateral weakness of hip abductor muscles (Myopathy / Muscular Dystrophy)
  - Antalgic Gait
- Is there limitation of the patient's range of movement? This can be reduced in chronic joint pathology (Osteoarthritis, inflammatory arthritis)

Inspection of the Spine

Although slightly counter-intuitive, when examining the spine it is important to inspect from anterior, lateral and posterior views to fully assess the patient.

Anterior inspection:

- Scars - anterior neck scar (anterior cervical discectomy)
- Posture - asymmetry, scoliosis
- Shoulder girdle asymmetry - scoliosis, fracture, dislocation, arthritis
- Pelvic tilt - scoliosis, abnormal leg length, hip abductor weakness

Lateral inspection:

- Cervical lordosis - hyperlordosis (chronic degenerative joint disease – OA)
- Thoracic kyphosis (20-45°) - hyperkyphosis (Scheurmann's Disease – congenital wedging of vertebrae)
- Lumbar lordosis – loss of lordosis (AS – sacroiliac joint dysfunction)
  - Could be lost in spondylolisthesis

Posterior inspection:

- Posture - asymmetry, scoliosis
  - In particular assess spinal alignment and Iliac crest alignment
- Skin + muscles = muscle wasting (paraspinals), scars, redness, bruising
- Soft tissue abnormalities: Lipomas, abnormal hair growth (occult spina bifida), Pigmentation, Café-au-lait spots (neurofibromatosis), Shagreen patches (tuberous sclerosis)

FEEL

Prior to palpation ensure to ask the patient about any pain. Palpate the following landmarks to assess for any tenderness, swelling or abnormal growths.

- Spinous processes + over sacroiliac joints – check for alignment + tenderness
- Paraspinal muscles – assess for tenderness + increased tone (spasms)
- Consider spinal percussion over thoracic/ lumbar spinous processes
  - Percussion tenderness is a sign of serious pathology (i.e., malignancy, osteomyelitis, compression fracture)

MOVE

As with any examination – it is important to assess both passive and active movements. When passively moving the joints ensure to place a hand over the joint to feel for crepitus. Assess the movements of the spine by giving the patient the following instructions:

Cervical spine:

- Flexion - tuck chin to chest; Normal Range of Movement (NROM) = 0-80°
- Extension - look up towards the ceiling; NROM = 0-50°
- Lateral flexion - try to touch your ear to your shoulder; NROM = 0-45°
- Rotation - look over your left/right shoulder; NROM = 0-80°

Thoracic spine:

- Rotation - ask the patient to sit on the side of bed + cross their arms across chest; twist the patient left + right as far as comfortable (stabilise hips if needed)

Lumbar spine:

- Flexion - touch toes whilst keeping legs straight
- Extension (10-20°) - lean back as far as comfortable
- Lateral flexion - slide hand down each leg

Special Tests

These tests can be used to find specific pathological signs linked to common or serious conditions affecting the spine.

Schober's Test

- Identifies restricted flexion of lumbar spine; occurs in inflammatory arthritis and ankylosing spondylitis
- Method:

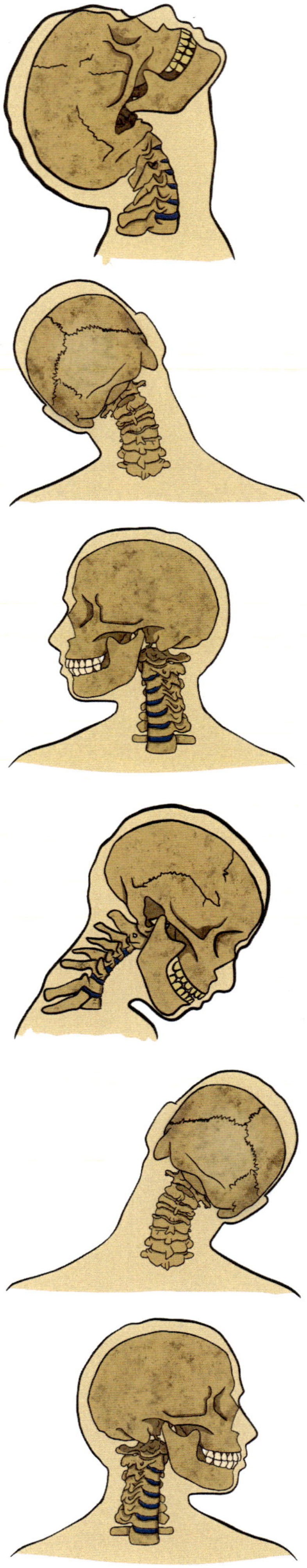

Cervical Spine Movements

- » Identify the location of posterior superior iliac spine (PSIS) on each side
- » Mark the skin at the midline point that lies 5cm below PSIS
- » Measure 15cm up from this point and mark the skin in the midline (10cm above PSIS)
- » Ask patient to touch their toes to assess lumbar flexion
- » Measure the distance between two lines (NORMAL = initial 15cm to >20cm)
- o <5cm difference implies lumbar flexion limitation that may be due to Ankylosing spondylitis if other symptoms are present.

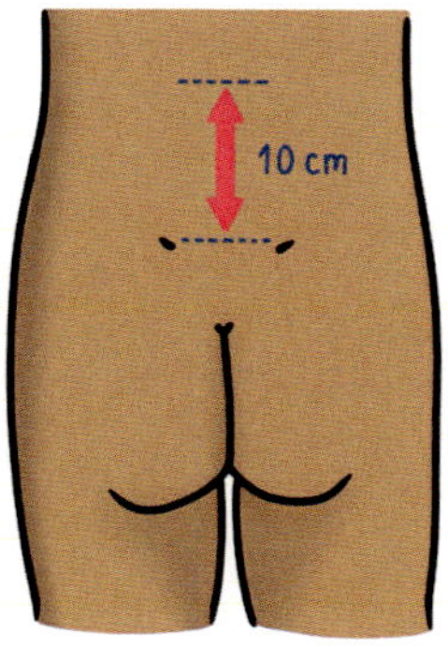

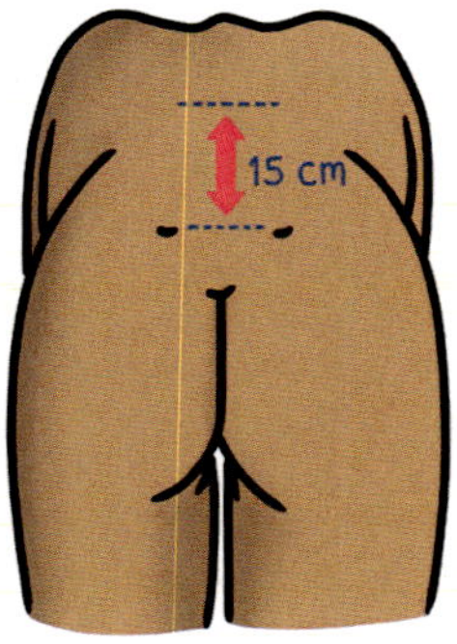

Adam's Forward Bend Test

- o Ask the patient to lean forward and observe for asymmetry in scapulae. When a patient has scoliosis, one side of their back is usually higher than the other. If a patient does not have scoliosis, their back appears straight.

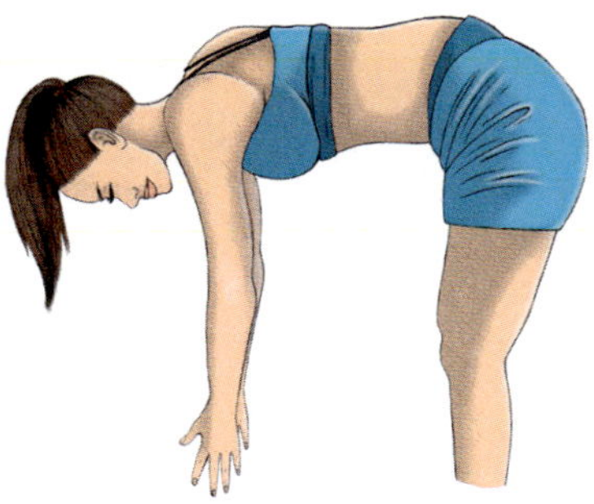

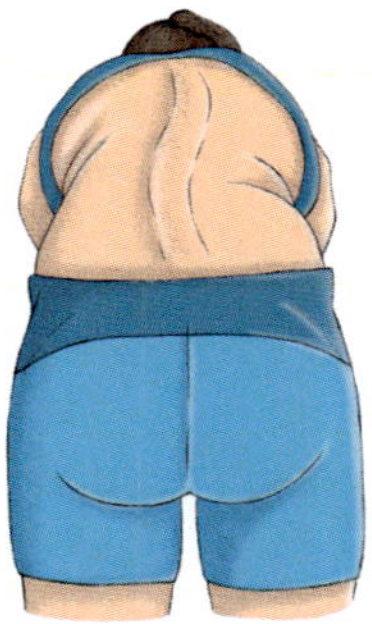

Chest circumference expansion = measure chest circumference in inspiration + expiration

- o Normal = 7cm difference
- o Abnormal = <5cm suggests Ankylosing Spondylitis

Femoral Nerve Stretch Test - identifies femoral nerve irritation

- o Position patient prone on the bed
- o Flex patient's knee to 90° then extend hip joint
- o Finally, plantarflex patient's foot
  - » If the patient experiences pain in their anterior thigh or inguinal region then this indicates femoral nerve irritation (usually secondary to L2-4 disc herniation).

Straight Leg Raise (Sciatic nerve stretch test; Lasegue's Sign) – assesses for sciatic nerve irritation

- o Position patient supine on the bed
- o Holding patient's ankle, raise their leg by passively flexing hip whilst keeping patient's knee fully extended
- o NROM passive hip flexion = 80-90°
- o Once patient's hip is flexed, dorsiflex patient's foot
  - » If the patient experiences pain in their posterior thigh or buttock, then this indicated sciatic nerve irritation (usually due to L4-S1 disc herniation / facet joint impingement)

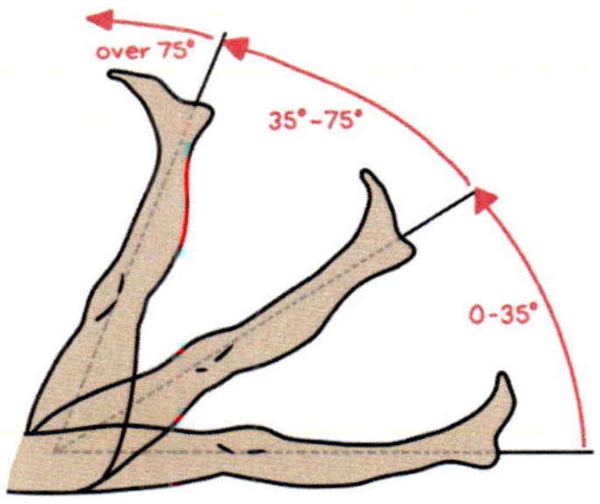

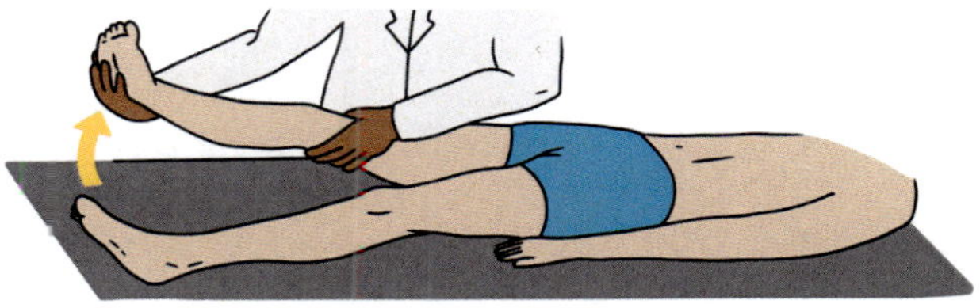

Gaenslen's Sacroiliac Stress Test – assesses for sacroiliac joint pathology

- o Ask the patient to flex their hip + knee, then passively push that knee into patient's chest whilst pushing contralateral thigh into bed
  - » If the patient experiences pain

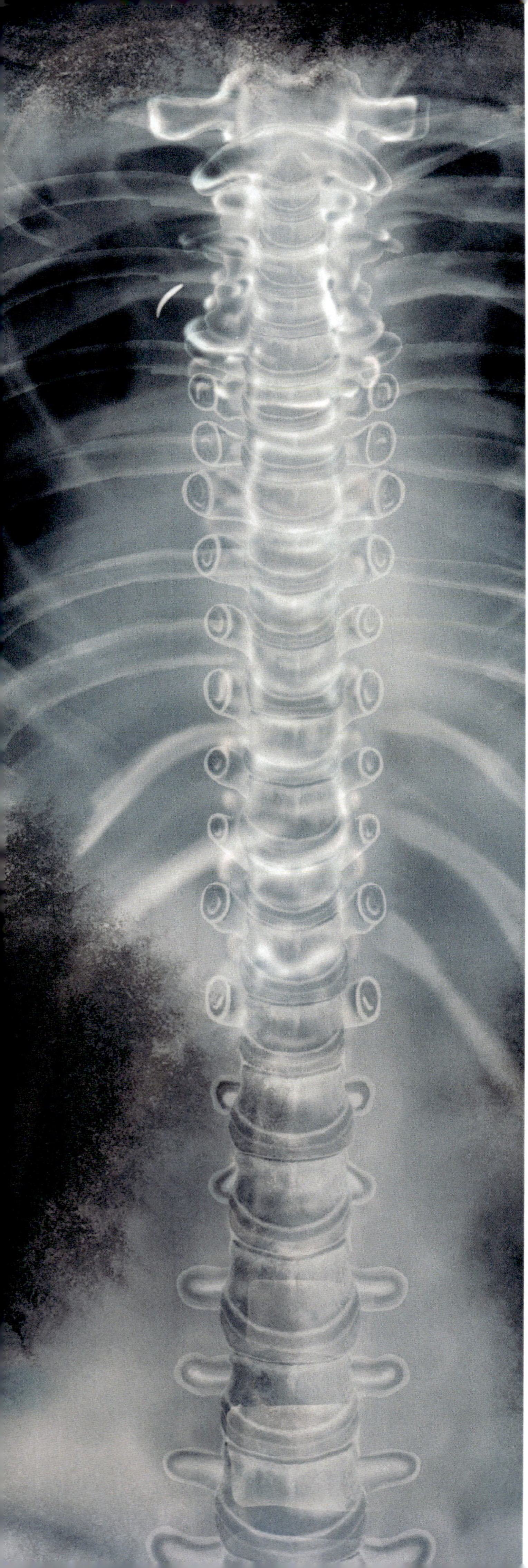

then this indicates a sacroiliac joint pathology

To complete an examination of the spine you can include neurological examinations of the upper and lower limbs if clinically relevant.

*Tip – it is important to examine the joints above and below the joint you have examined.

In an OSCE scenario in particular – to complete a full spinal examination, you should state that you would examine the hip and shoulder joints, perform a full neurovascular examination of the upper and lower limbs, perform a PR exam to test perianal sensation & anal tone, and request further imaging if necessary (X-Ray/MRI).

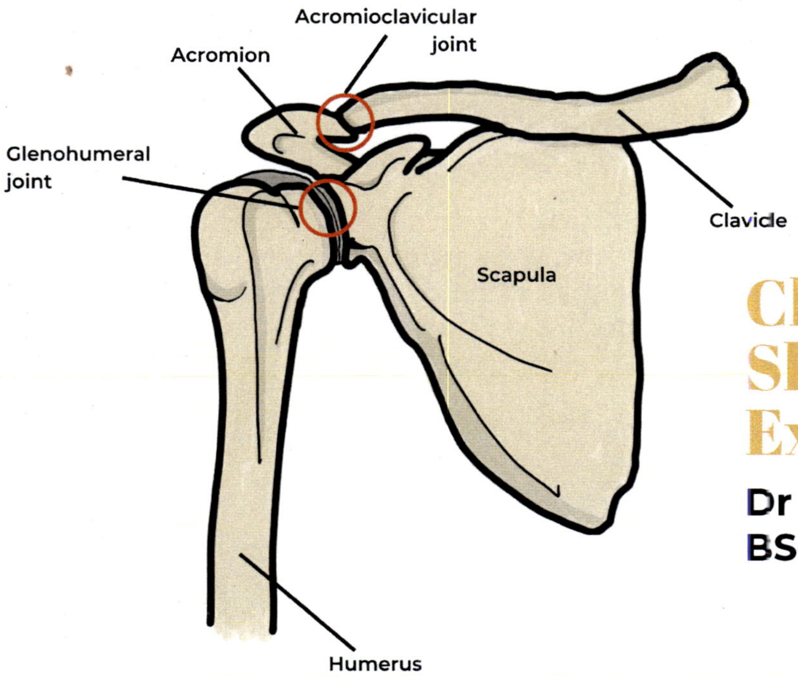

Chapter 3: Shoulder Examination

Dr Katriona Hutchison
BSc MBChB

The shoulder 'joint' is composed of two separate joints: the glenohumeral joint and the acromioclavicular joint. Three bones are involved in these joints: the humerus, the acromion (of the scapula) and the clavicle. A series of muscles and ligaments serve to stabilize the joint and allow movement.

The shoulder joint is a ball and socket joint and allows the following movements: flexion, extension, abduction, adduction, and rotation. When examining the shoulder joint it is essential to assess all these movements in turn.

As with all examinations, prior to examining the patient, you should introduce yourself, confirm the patient's name and date of birth, explain what the examination entails and gain patient consent. Before starting the examination check with the patient if they have any pain in their shoulders.

LOOK

Begin with a general inspection – assess if the patient is comfortable or appears to be in pain. Are they wearing a brace or sling? Do they appear to be cradling one side in protection?

When examining the shoulders, you need to expose both shoulder joints and ask the patient to stand or sit up straight.

Inspect the shoulders looking from the front, back and sides.

What to look for on inspection?

- Symmetry Vs Deformity
  - Do the shoulders look symmetrical both anteriorly and posteriorly?
  - Is there any deformity or loss of contour?
- Winging
  - Look at the shoulders from the back to assess for any winging of the scapula.
- Skin Changes
  - Are there any wounds, scars, sinuses, bruising or swelling?
- Muscle Wasting
  - Look at the large muscle groups associated with the shoulder including deltoid and the rotator cuff muscles (supraspinatus, infraspinatus, subscapularis and teres minor) for any sign of wasting.

FEEL

When palpating the shoulder joints, ensure to compare the two joints with every step and check with the patient throughout for any pain.

- Temperature
  - Use the back of your hand and assess temperature of the skin anteriorly, posteriorly and superiorly to the joint.

- Palpate the bony processes involved in the shoulder joints:
  - Start at the sternoclavicular joint and palpate along the clavicle to the acromioclavicular joint. Don't forget to palpate the coracoid process (sits inferior to the lateral aspect of the clavicle)
  - Palpate the acromion, along the spine of scapula before returning laterally to palpate the head of the humerus.
- Palpate the anterior and posterior joint lines
- Palpate the large muscle groups
  - Deltoid, supraspinatus and infraspinatus
- Assess sensation through light touch of the 'regimental badge' area (lateral superior aspect of upper arm). This area is innervated by the axillary nerve.

MOVE

When moving any joint it is important to test passive and active movement. Passive movement will allow an examiner to assess muscle tone, to feel for crepitus, and to assess movement of the joint without active input from the patient. To assess passive movement of a joint, place one hand over the joint and use the other to hold the limb at the distal extremity. This will enable you to direct the limb in different directions to assess all planes of movement.

At the shoulder joint **passively** assess the following movements from the anatomical position:

- Flexion – raise arm anteriorly (forward) away from the body
- Extension – Take arm posteriorly (backward) as far back as the patient is able
- Abduction (away from the midline) – raise arm outwards and upwards
- Adduction (towards the midline) – move arm towards and across the body keeping the elbow straight and their hand at waist level
- External Rotation – bend elbows and tuck them into the side of the body. Move the patient's hands away from the midline whilst keeping the elbows fixed against their sides.
- Internal Rotation – abduct arm with a bent elbow and fingers pointing towards the floor, then take the patient's hand across their back.

Now ask the patients to repeat the above movements independently **(active)**. Assess for any difficulty or pain experienced when attempting the above normal movements of the shoulder.

*Tip – when assessing active internal rotation you can ask the patient to try to touch their shoulder blades from their lower back.

Common Pathologies

Most examinations of the shoulder will not elicit any signs but particular signs to look out for and their associated pathologies are detailed below:

Frozen Shoulder

- Stiff and painful shoulder with consequent reduced range of movement. Patients present with acute onset pain followed by long-term stiffness which tends to last 18-24 months before starting to resolve.
- Key signs – External rotation is <50% of their baseline, pain and reduced range of movement in abduction.

Dislocations

- Anterior Shoulder Dislocation – occurs secondary to trauma (often from a fall onto an out-stretched hand). On examination there is a loss of the shoulder contour – deltoid muscle appears flattened.
  - Always assess sensation of the lateral surface of the upper arm (regimental badge area) as anterior dislocations are often associated with axillary nerve palsy and consequent loss of sensation in this area.
- Posterior Shoulder Dislocation – uncommon injury. Characterised by limitation of external rotation in both active and passive examination.

Rotator Cuff Injury

- Painful shoulder and reduced range of movement secondary to trauma or degeneration.
- Key signs: Shoulder weakness and pain on abduction. If complete tear then patient may be completely unable to abduct arm. If the examiner passively abducts the arm >15 degrees from the midline then the patient may be able to hold it in place through use of the deltoid (major muscle in abduction after first 15 degrees).

Impingement Syndrome

- Impingement of the supraspinatus tendon as it runs through the subacromial space secondary to subacromial tendinopathy or acromioclavicular joint osteoarthritis
- Key sign on examination: pain and reduced range of movement particularly in abduction. Known as the painful arc where patient experiences pain when abducting the arm 60-120 degrees from the midline.

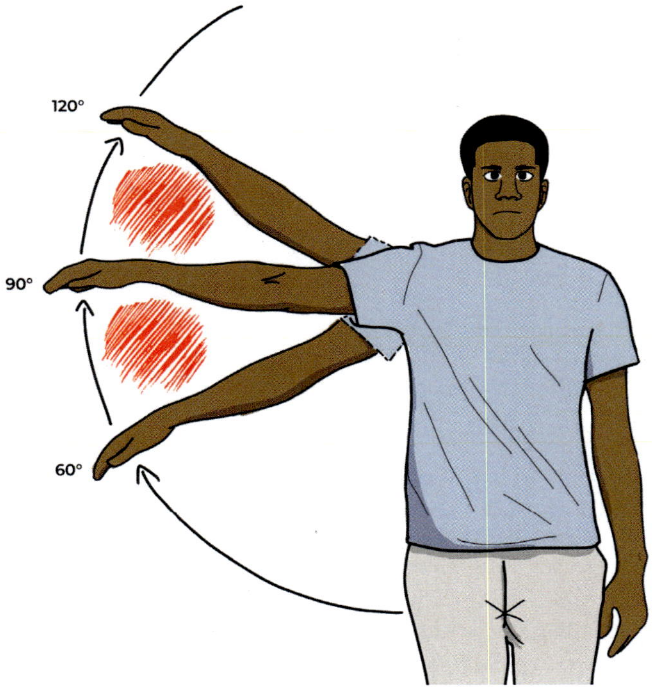

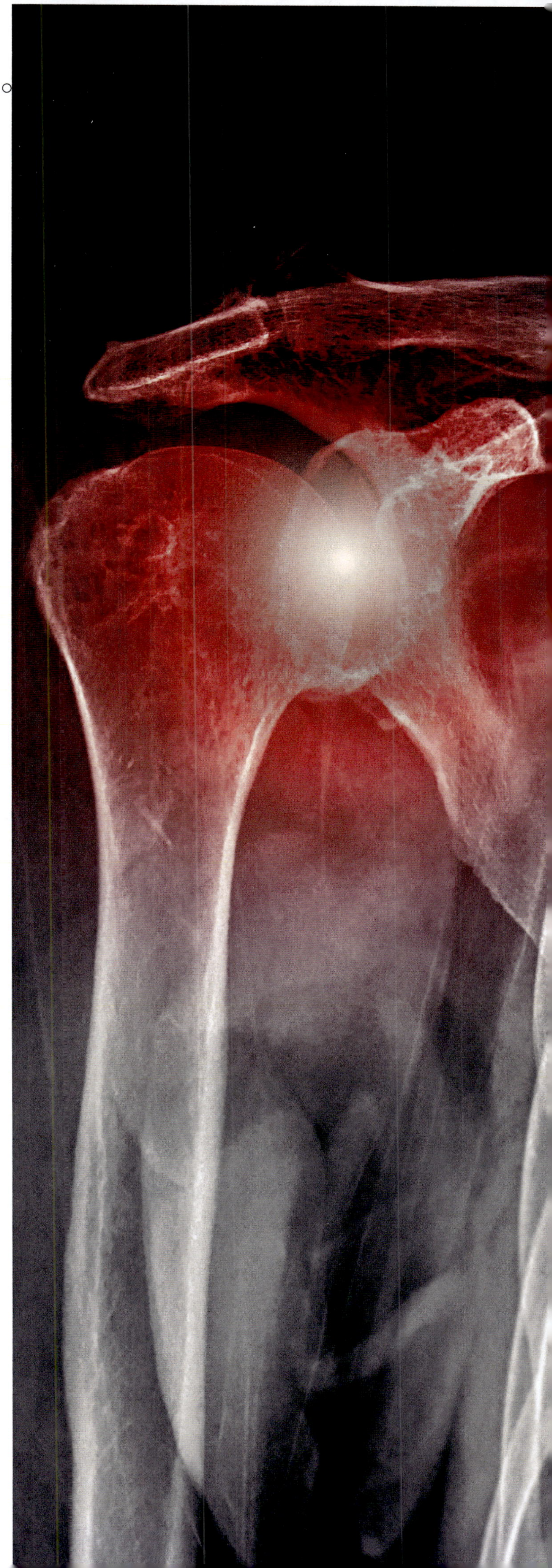

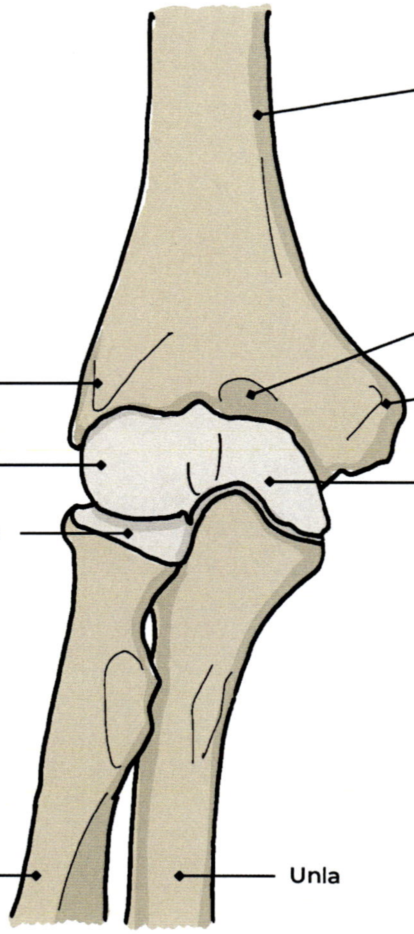

Chapter 4: Elbow Examination

Dr Riya Thomas MbChB

The elbow joint is a hinge joint composed of three bones: the humerus, ulna, and radius. These form two articulations: humero-ulnar; between the trochlea of the humerus and trochlear notch of the ulna, and humero-radial; between capitulum and upper surface of radial head. Although not considered part the elbow joint, the proximal radioulnar joint (as the name describes), exists between the proximal aspects of the radius and ulna, and is a pivot joint.

In the anatomical position, the carrying angle, or the natural valgus angle of the elbow, it is normally around 5 - 15 degrees. Movements of the elbow include flexion and extension and the elbow joint itself, whilst pronation and supination are movements that occur at the proximal and distal radioulnar joints.

Prior to beginning your examination of the elbow ensure to introduce yourself to the patient, confirm the patient's name and date of birth, explain the examination and gain consent. Ensure the patient's upper limbs are adequately exposed to the shoulders, and they are standing with their arms positioned in the anatomical position.

LOOK

On inspection it is important to visualise both elbow joints from the front, back, and sides.

General inspection

- Does the patient appear comfortable?
- Look around the patient for: mobility aids, slings.

Deformity

- Assess the Carrying Angle
  - A carrying angle >15° is known as Cubitus valgus. This may be a congenital deformity or associated with previous trauma.
  - A carrying angle of <5° is known as Cubitus varus ("gunstock" deformity). This can occur as a complication of supracondylar fracture of the humerus.
- Fixed flexion deformity
  - Can be caused by previous trauma or muscle spasticity

Skin changes

- Psoriasis, scars, erythema

Swelling

- Assess for intra- and extra-articular swellings
- May indicate joint effusion, trauma, or inflammatory arthropathy

Muscles

- "Popeye" sign indicates a biceps tendon rupture
- Inspect for signs of muscle wasting

FEEL

Ask about pain before starting palpation of any joint. Ensure to compare each movement between the two elbows.

Temperature

- Using the bank of your hands, assess for any difference in temperature over the arm, elbow joint and forearm; compare with the other side.

Palpate the bony prominences

- Olecranon
  - Pain and swelling can suggest bursitis
- Medial and lateral epicondyle
  - Pain on palpation of medical epicondyle may suggest medical epicondylitis (Golfer's elbow)
  - Pain on palpation of lateral epicondyle may suggest lateral epicondylitis (Tennis elbow)
- Radial head – palpate whilst rotating the forearm into supine and prone positions.

Bend elbow to 90° to assess for any effusion

Palpate the biceps tendon

- Ask the patient to actively flex their elbow to 90° and feel for the biceps tendon anteriorly over the joint

MOVE

The movements of the elbow joint should be assessed and compared with the opposite side. Both active and passive movement should be examined.

Active movement

- Elbow extension (0°) – ask the patient to stretch their arms in front of them, as straight as they can.
- Elbow flexion (145°)– from the above position, ask the patient to bend their elbows to touch their shoulders
- Pronation (90°)– with their elbow held at 90° flexion, ask the patient to turn their forearm so that their palm is facing downwards.
- Supination (90°) – ask the patient to turn their forearm so that their palm is facing upwards.

Passive movement

- Allow the patient to relax their arm and repeat the above movements passively
- Feel for crepitus at the joint whilst assessing passive movements
  - When assessing for pronation/ supination you should be palpating the proximal radioulnar joint to feel for crepitus

Common Signs on Elbow Examination

- Medial epicondylitis (Golfer's elbow) – inflammation at the common insertion site of the flexor tendons due overuse
  - Pain on palpation of the bony prominence of the medical epicondyle
  - Pain can be reproduced with resisted wrist flexion
  - Absence of warmth, erythema, or swelling (as with other causes of acute inflammation)
- Lateral epicondylitis (Tennis elbow) – inflammation at the common insertion point of the extensor tendons due to overuse.
  - Pain on palpation around the lateral epicondyle
  - Pain can be reproduced with resisted wrist extension
  - Absence of warmth, erythema, or swelling (as with other causes of acute inflammation)
- Olecranon bursitis – inflammation of the olecranon bursa, a fluid filled pouch which lies over the olecranon process. Inflammation may be caused

by repeated trauma, infection, or other inflammatory process (e.g. inflammatory arthropathy)

- Obvious swelling over the olecranon process, fluctuant in nature
- Pain only on full flexion of the elbow joint
- Range of movement is usually preserved
- Abrasions or overlying skin changes may be present if infective cause
- Warmth, erythema, and pain on palpation of the bursa if infective cause

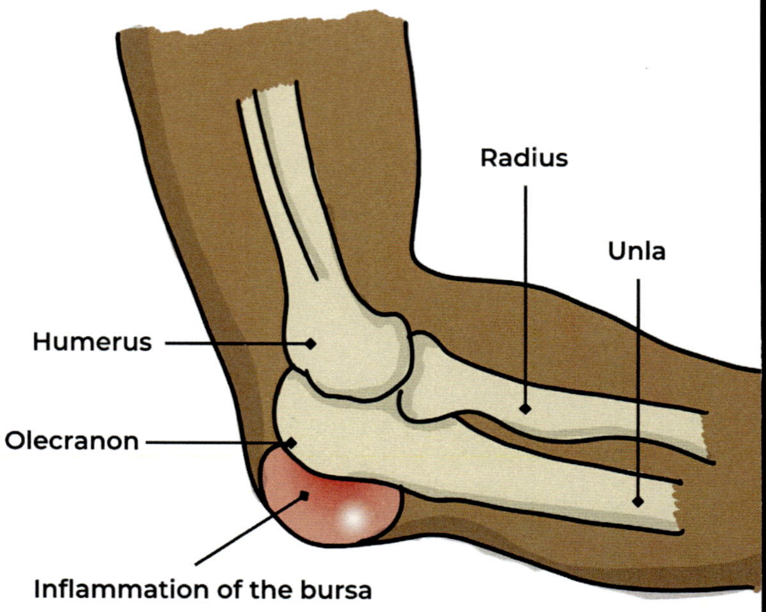

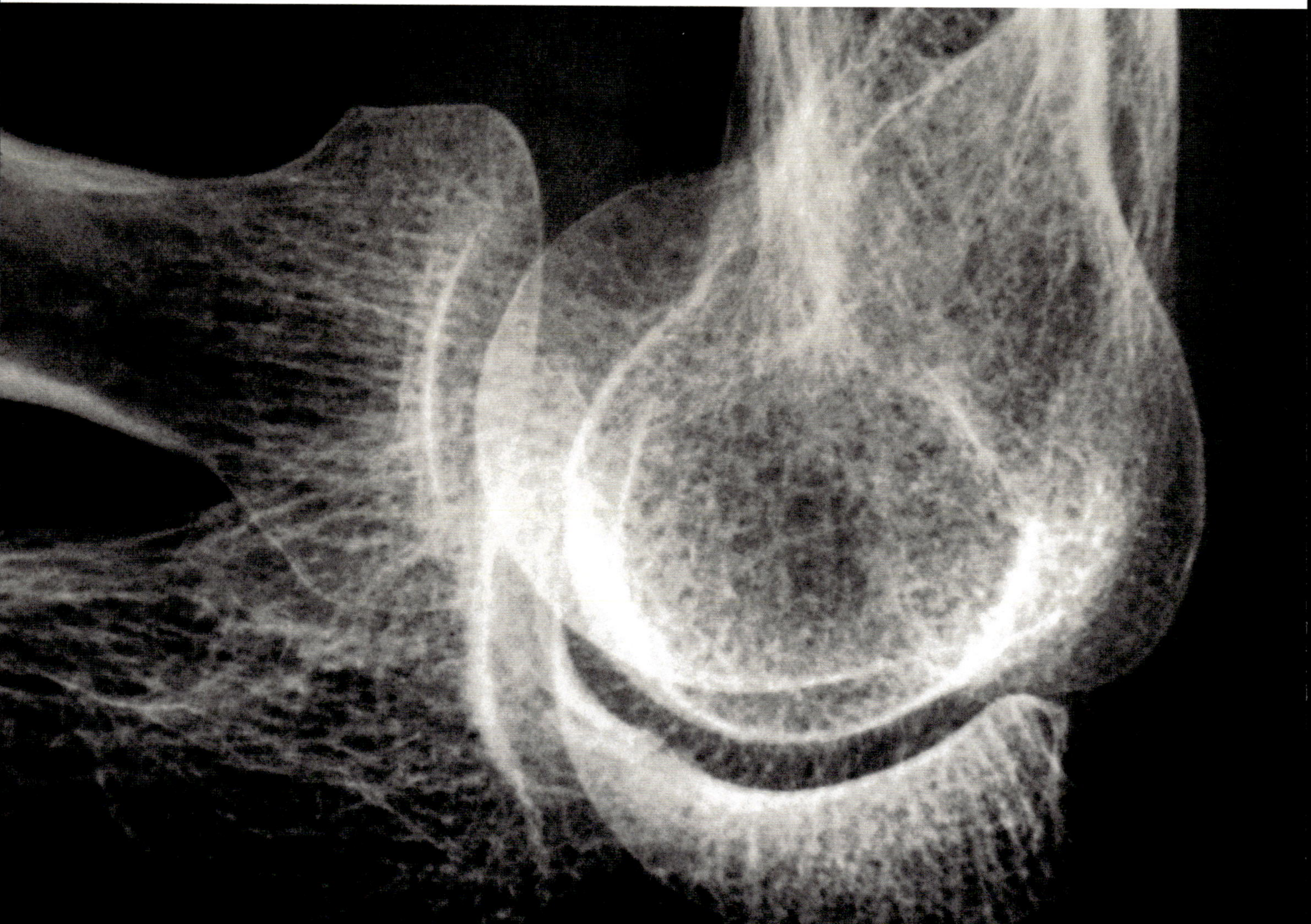

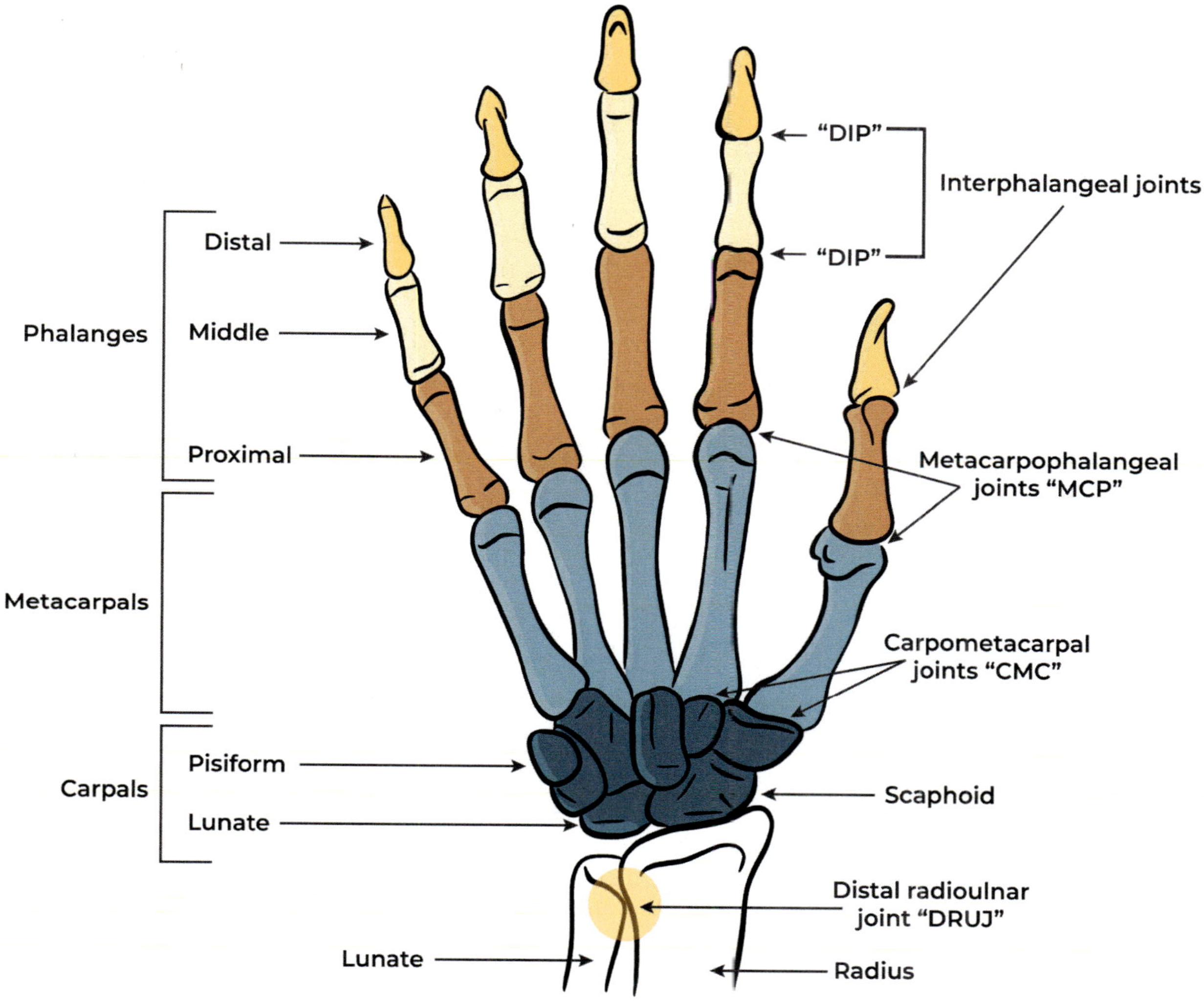

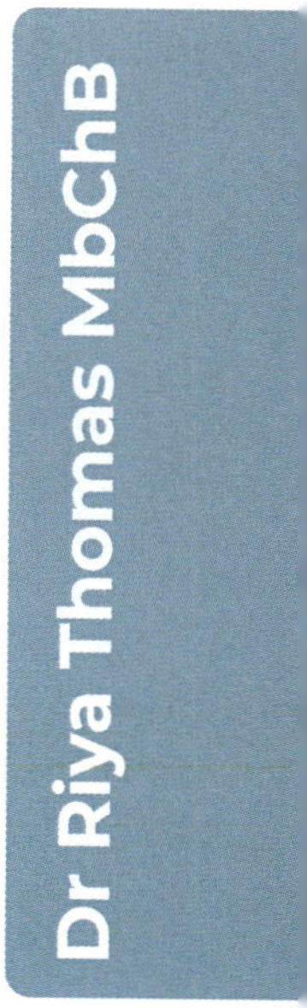

Chapter 5: Wrist & Hand Examination

Dr Riya Thomas MbChB

The anatomy of the wrist and hand comprises many different functional joints. The wrist joint consists of the distal articular surface of the radius and the carpal bones. There are eight carpal bones arranged in two rows: scaphoid, lunate, triquetrum, pisiform, trapezium, trapezoid, capitate, and hamate. The carpometacarpal (CMC) joints connect the carpals to the five metacarpals. Distally, the metacarpophalangeal (MCP) joints then allow movement of the phalanges. The proximal (PIP) and distal (DIP) interphalangeal joints allow flexion with minimal extension.

Important muscles of the hand include the thenar muscles, located at the base of the thumb with a bulge (the thenar eminence), and the hypothenar muscles, on the medial side of the palm which form the hypothenar eminence.

The carpal tunnel is an osseo-fibrous space on the palmar aspect of the wrist, which serves as a passageway to the palm for flexor tendons and the median nerve. The median, radial, and ulnar nerves provide sensation to the hand and wrist.

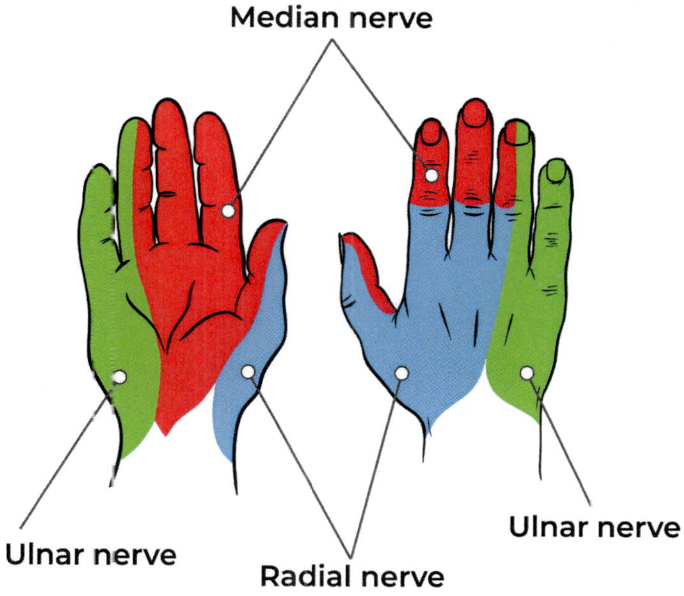

Prior to your examination, introduce yourself to the patient, confirm the patient's name and date of birth, explain the examination and gain consent. Ensure the hands and arms are adequately exposed to the elbows. Begin with the patient sitting, and with their hands resting in front of them on a pillow.

LOOK

General inspection

- Does the patient appear comfortable?
- Look around the patient for any splints.

Inspect the dorsal surface then the palmar surface of the hand

- Dorsum
  - Nail changes – pitting, onycholysis
  - Skin – scars, rashes, or erythema
  - Deformity
    - "Swan neck" and boutonnière deformity secondary to rheumatoid arthritis
    - Ulnar deviation at the wrist
    - Heberden's nodes at the DIP joints and Bouchard's nodes at PIP joints secondary to osteoarthritis.
  - Swelling – ganglions
- Palmar
  - Skin – erythema, scars (e.g. carpal tunnel release scar)
  - Deformity – Dupuytren's contracture causing fingers to bend toward the palm
  - Swellings – ganglions
  - Muscle wasting – thenar wasting indicates a median nerve lesion

FEEL

Always ask if the patient has any pain before starting any palpation. Ensure to compare each step with the opposite wrist and hand.

Temperature

- Using the back of your hand, assess and compare the temperature of the forearm, the dorsal aspect of wrist, the MCP joints and the phalanges.

Pulses

- Palpate the radial and ulnar pulses
- Measure the capillary refill in the fingertips

Palpate the bulk of the thenar and hypothenar eminences to assess for wasting

Nerve sensation

- Test median nerve sensation over the thenar eminence or index finger
- Test ulnar nerve sensation over hypothenar eminence or little finger
- Test radial nerve sensation over the dorsal web space between thumb and index finger or anatomical snuffbox

MCP joint squeeze

- Gently squeeze over the row of MCP joints whilst observing the patient for signs of discomfort

Bimanual palpation – using your thumbs, squeeze across the joints from distal to proximal, feeling for tenderness or bony swellings

- Distal radio-ulnar joint
- Radiocarpal joint
- MCP Joints
- PIP Joints
- DIP Joints
- CMC Joint of the thumb

Palpate the anatomical snuffbox

- Tenderness in this location suggests a scaphoid fracture

MOVE

The movements of the wrist and hand joints in each arm should be assessed and compared. Assess both active and passive movement.

Wrist movements

- Extension – ask the patient to put the palms of their hands together, making a "prayer" sign
- Flexion – ask the patient to put the backs of their hands together, making a "reverse prayer" sign

Finger movements

- Flexion – ask the patient to make a fist
- Extension and abduction – ask the patient to open up their first and spread their fingers out

Thumb movements

- Abduction – ask the patient to point their thumb to the ceiling, with their wrist supinated
- Opposition – ask the patient to touch their thumb to their little finger tip

Passive movement

- Repeat the above movements passively, feel for any crepitus as you move the joint

Assess motor function

- Radial nerve – test wrist extension; ask the patient to stretch their arms out in front of them with their palms facing down, then ask them to cock their wrists back. Ask them to keep their wrists cocked back whilst you apply resistance.
- Ulnar nerve – test finger abduction against resistance; ask the patient to spread their fingers out and stop you from pushing them together
- Median nerve – assess thumb abduction; ask the patient to point their thumbs to the ceiling with the palms facing up, ask them to keep this position whilst you try to push their thumb down

Common Signs on Wrist and Hand Examination

- Rheumatoid arthritis (RA) – the following findings in the hands occur as a result of RA
  - Swan neck deformity: PIP joint hyperextension + DIP joint flexion
  - Boutonnière: PIP joint flexion + DIP joint hyperextension
  - Z-thumb: IP joint hyperextension + MCP joint flexion
  - Ulnar deviation
- Dupuytren's contracture – thickening of the palmar fascia which causes one or more fingers to curl in towards the palm, preventing finger extension.
- Carpal tunnel syndrome – narrowing of the carpal tunnel which compresses the median nerve
  - Patients present with tingling or pain in the thumb, index, and middle fingers, wasting of thenar muscles and reduced sensation over the radial three and a half digits

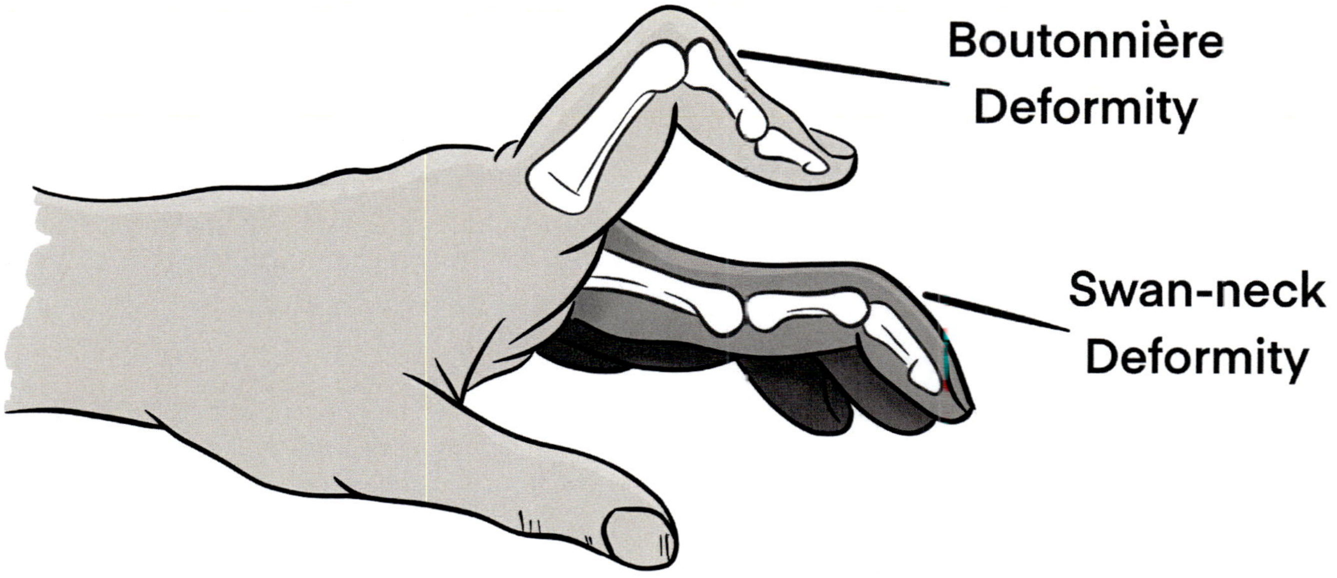

Chapter 6: Hip Examination

Dr Barrie Lyell
BSc (Hons) MBChB

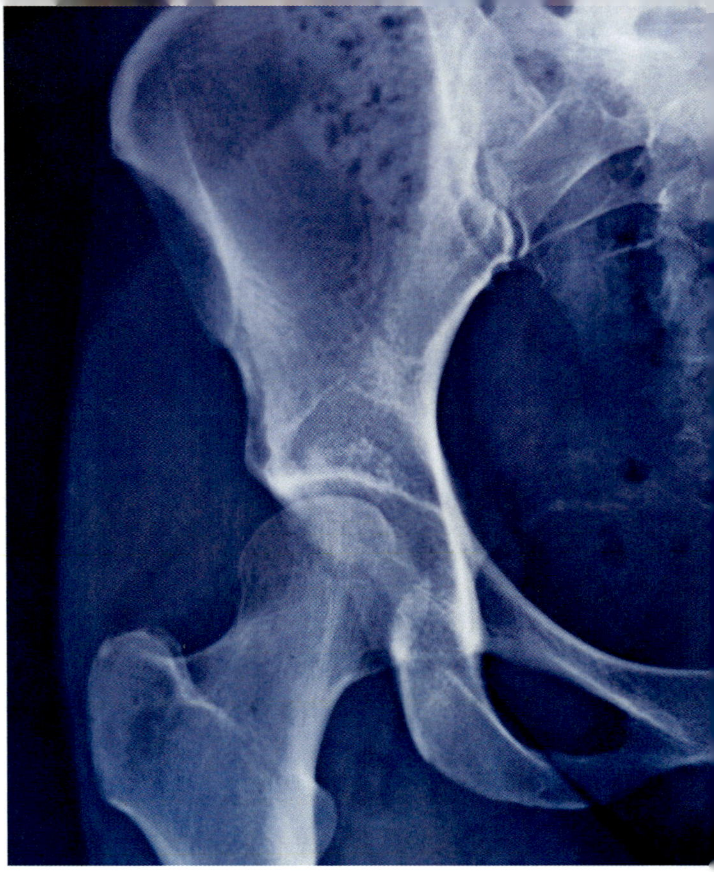

The hip is a ball and socket joint made up of the acetabulum of the pelvis and the head of the femur. Ball and socket joints enable a multitude of movements around a central axis. These movements are flexion, extension, abduction, adduction, internal rotation and external rotation.

As with all examinations begin with an introduction, confirming the patient's name and date of birth, give an explanation of the examination and obtain patient consent. Prior to starting the examination – enquire if the patient has any pain or has had any recent surgery to the joint.

Expose both legs fully but maintain modesty where possible (in clinical practice you may need to see the entire hip joint and gluteal muscle mass).

LOOK

General Inspection

- Inspect the bedspace for any mobility aids
- Look at the drug chart for analgesia, bisphosphonates, calcium/Vit D supplements, or biologics

Ask the patient to lie down on the bed and look for the following signs:

- Signs of pain or discomfort e.g. grimacing, clutching joint
- Signs of systemic infection which may suggest a septic joint e.g. sweating, flushing, rigors
- Body habitus: obesity is a significant risk factor for osteoarthritis, cachexia which could be associated with bony metastases
- Obvious joint pathology in joints other than the hips e.g. hand and finger deformities associated with rheumatoid arthritis
- Shortened and externally rotated hip – classical sign of a neck of femur fracture as the short external rotators act on the joint

Ask the patient to stand to examine the following features:

- Malalignment of the legs, looking for any tilting of the pelvis. Assess from both the front and the back of the patient.
- Gluteal muscle wasting. The gluteal muscle is quick to atrophy, and due to its large size, even relatively small differences in size are easily noted.
- Quadriceps wasting.
- Swelling or redness of the joint itself. However, the hip joint is relatively deep so external signs of inflammation may not always be present.
- Scars, usually on the lateral aspect, which may indicate previous surgery or trauma.

FEEL

Begin by assessing the patient in the supine position with legs straight (hips not flexed).

Temperature

- Feel for temperature changes above and below the joint using the back of the hand; this may indicate inflammatory or septic arthritis.

Palpate the Greater Trochanter

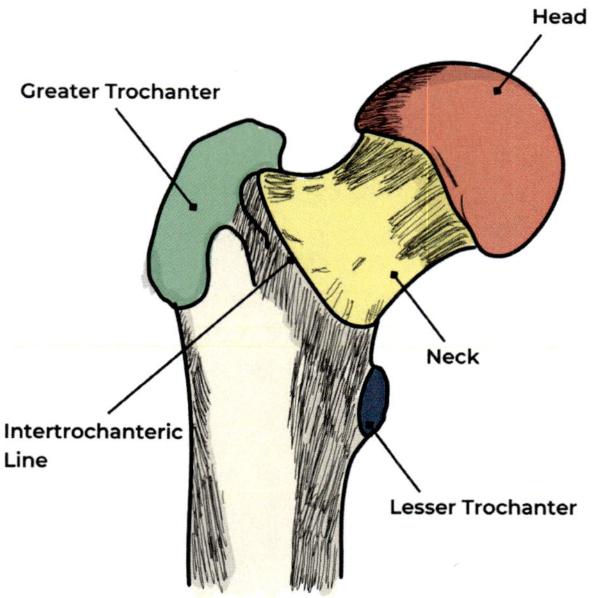

- Palpation of the hip joint is limited due to the deep nature of the joint.
- The greater trochanter is located at the lateral aspect of the hip joint. Pain on palpation of the greater trochanter may indicate trochanteric bursitis.

Measure for Leg Length Discrepancy

- Apparent Leg Length Discrepancy – measure from the xiphisternum to each medial malleoli to assess for any difference in length
  - Known as apparent as not due to actual leg length discrepancy but rather is secondary to pelvic tilt.
- True Leg Length Discrepancy – measure from the anterior superior iliac spine (ASIS) to the medial malleolus of the same leg. Repeat on the opposite side.
  - This will show if there is an actual leg length discrepancy; this can be congenital, or acquired secondary to trauma or degenerative disease

MOVE

Assess for both ACTIVE (patient moving joint) and PASSIVE (examiner moving joint) movement. Check for pain throughout the examination by keeping a close eye on the patient's facial expressions. During passive movement remember to keep one hand on the hip joint to feel for crepitus.

Flexion

- Active: Ask the patient to bring their knee towards their head as far as they can (hip flexion). Remember! Flexion of the lumbar spine and pelvis may contribute to an appearance of hip flexion; this can be assessed by placing a hand under the lumbar spine and checking for loss of lordosis.
- Passive: assess for passive hip flexion by supporting the weight of the lower limb and bringing their knee towards their head, noting any differences from active flexion.
- Normal angle of maximum flexion is 110°

Extension

- Most accurately done with the patient in the prone position, but can be assessed with the patient lying on their side (the opposite side to the joint being examined). Usually in an OSCE you would only need to offer this.
- Active: with patient lying prone ask them to keep their leg straight and lift their ankle off the ground
- Passive: whilst holding the patient's ankle, gently lift the limb off the bed.
- Normal extension is 10-20°.

Internal and External Rotation

- Active: Ask patient to bend their knee then move it medially and laterally.
- Passive: Using both hands, roll the patient's thigh internally and externally whilst still on the bed. With the hip and knee both flexed to 90°, internally

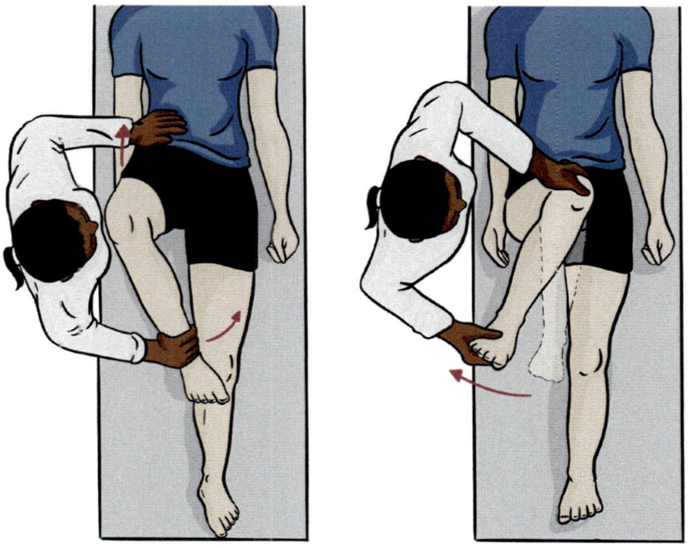

and externally rotate the hip as illustrated in the picture below.

- Normal range of motion is 45° of both internal and external rotation.

Abduction and Adduction

- To control for tilting of the pelvis during active examination place one hand on their contralateral ASIS. Lean your other forearm on their right ASIS.
- Active: ask the patient to keep their leg straight and move it sideways away from their body, and then to the other side crossing over the other leg.
- Passive: whilst your left hand stabilises the contralateral ASIS, passively abduct the right lower limb away from the midline with your right hand. Then use your right hand to stabilise the ipsilateral ASIS and adduct the limb across the midline in front over the opposite leg. Repeat these steps for the other leg.

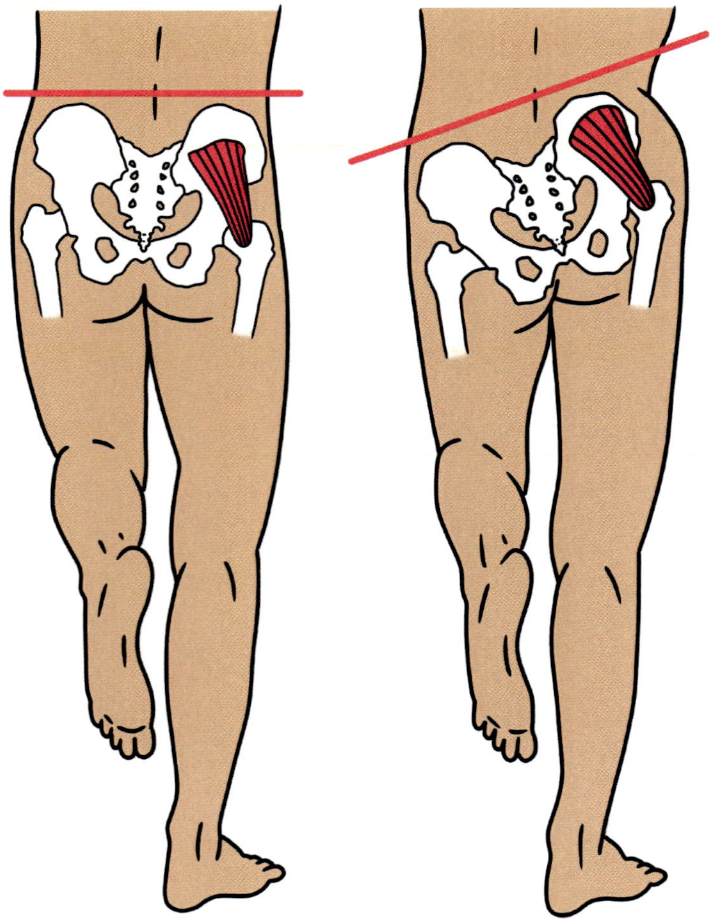

Trendelenburg's Gait

» Normal abduction is 45° and adduction is 30°.

Special Tests

Trendelenburg Sign

- Ask the patient to stand on one leg, ensuring you are nearby and ready to support them in case of loss of balance. Trendelenburg Sign is positive if the pelvis dips to the side that is opposite to the leg the patient is standing on. This is usually a sign of weak hip abductors on the side of the standing leg.

Thomas' Test

- Place your hand, palm up, underneath the patient's lumbar spine. If assessing the right leg, ask the patient to bring their left knee towards their chest. The test is positive if at the point the lumbar lordosis is flattened, they are unable to keep their right leg flat on the bed. It tests for flexion contracture of the hip as seen in arthritis or certain neuromuscular disorders.

Ensure you have examined both hip joints and compared them throughout. Subsequently, assess the patient's gait for signs of Trendelenburg dip, an ataxic gait, or an antalgic gait.

To complete your examination, offer to examine the ipsilateral knee and lumbar spine (the joints below and above) to assess if the pain is referred. Additionally, for completeness, offer to perform a neurological exam of the lower limbs.

Conclude your examination by thanking the patient, summarizing your findings and recommending further investigations if applicable.

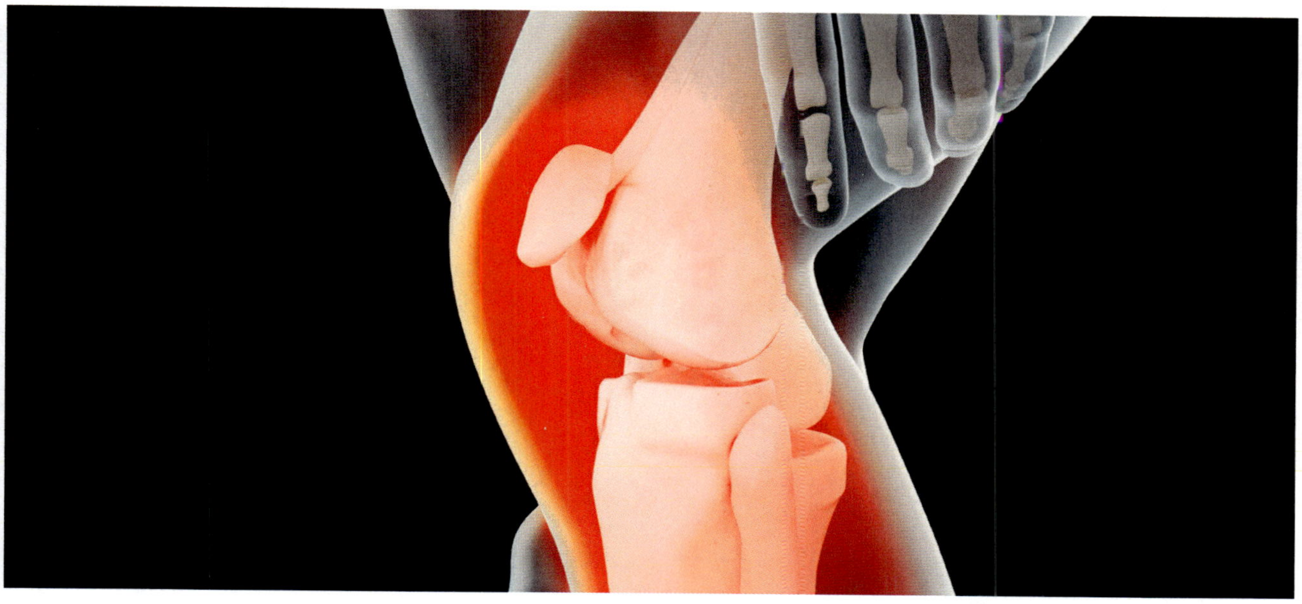

Chapter 7: Knee Examination

Dr Barrie Lyell BSc (Hons) MBChB

The knee is a hinge joint made up of 3 bones: the femur, tibia and patella. The knee joint consists of two articulations: tibiofemoral and patellofemoral. The tibiofemoral articulation exists between the medial and lateral condyles of the femur and the tibial condyles, whilst the patellofemoral articulation exists between the anterior aspect of the distal femur and the patella. The knee as a hinge joint, allows two key movements: flexion and extension. The knee also allows a small degree of medial and lateral rotation, but this is not assessed during examination.

As with all joint examinations, introduce yourself, wash your hands, confirm patient name and date of birth, explain the examination and obtain consent. Prior to examination, enquire about any pain or recent surgery affecting the knee or adjacent joints.

LOOK

To adequately examine the knee ask the patient to expose the knees, quadriceps and lower legs, whilst maintaining modesty where able.

Whilst the patient is exposing the knee joints watch the patient for any pain on movement. Inspect the bedspace for any mobility aids and look at the drug chart (if one is present) for any relevant medications (analgesia, bisphosphonates, calcium/vitamin D supplements, biologics).

Start by examining the patient whilst lying on the examination table – observe for the following signs:

- Signs of pain or discomfort e.g. grimacing, clutching joint
- Signs of systemic infection which may suggest a septic joint e.g. sweating, flushing, rigors
- Body habitus: obesity is a significant risk factor for osteoarthritis, cachexia could be associated with bony metastases
- Obvious joint pathology outside of the knee joints e.g. hand and finger deformities associated with rheumatoid arthritis

Then examine the patient whilst standing, assess the knee joint from the front, side, and the back of the patient looking for the following signs:

- Malalignment of the legs, looking for valgus (“knock knees”) or varus (“bow legs”) deformity. Assess from the front, side, and the back of the patient.
- Quadriceps muscle wasting - the quadriceps muscle is quick to atrophy, and due to its large size, even relatively small differences in size are easily noted. If suspected, measure the thigh circumference 10cm above the superior margin of the patella on both legs.
- Swelling or redness of the joint itself

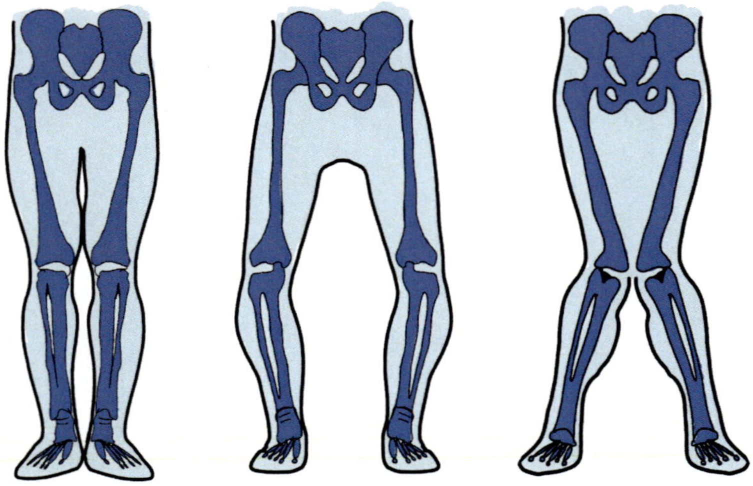

which may suggest a septic joint or inflammatory arthritis.

- Scars, which may indicate previous surgery or trauma.

FEEL

Ensure the patient is lying comfortably (bed at ~45°), and knees are extended.

Temperature

- Use the back of your hand to feel for warmth over the joint, as well as above and below the joint, and compare to the contralateral side.

Palpate for effusion

- Apply pressure to the patient's mid-thigh and move the pressure downwards towards the patella to empty the suprapatellar bursa. Keeping this hand in place, 'tap' the patella with the other hand. If a palpable or audible 'knock' of the patella on the femoral condyles is observed, this suggests a joint effusion (in the absence of pathology the patella should be in contact with the femoral condyles and therefore no 'knock' would be seen/ heard).
- Smaller effusions may be elicited my applying pressure on the medial side of the knee, running it in an upward direction medially, and then a downward direction laterally, looking for a 'bulge' on the medial side when pressure has shifted to the lateral side. If a bulge is present this is suggestive of an effusion.

Palpate the knee joint

- With the knee in 90° flexion and foot flat on the bed, use both hands to palpate over tibial tuberosity, patellar tendon, the margins of the patella, and the quadriceps tendon.
  - Pain on palpation of, or interruption to, the quadriceps tendon, suggests a problem with the extensor mechanism.
- Palpate medial and lateral joint lines for tenderness which may suggest meniscal pathology.
- Palpate behind the knee for tenderness or swellings e.g. Baker's cyst.

MOVE

When assessing movement in the joint assess both passively and actively. Use the following instructions to direct the patients in performing active movements.

Extension

- Ask the patient to lie their leg flat on the bed and fully tighten their quads to straighten their leg. Note any hyper-extension. With their leg straight, ask them to lift their leg off the bed to demonstrate that the extensor mechanism is intact.

Flexion

- Active: Ask patient to bring their foot towards their buttocks.
- Passive: See if any more flexion is possible by placing one hand on their knee, the other on their tibia, and attempting to flex the knee further.

Straighten the leg, keeping your hand on their knee to observe for crepitus.

Following assessment of flexion and extension it is important to assess the ligaments of the knee and if there are any abnormal movements of the knee joint secondary to trauma of the ligaments.

Anterior Cruciate Ligament (ACL) – Anterior Drawer Test

- With the knee in 90° flexion and foot flat on the bed, explain to the patient you are going to gently sit on their foot (enquire about foot pain first!). Gripping their upper tibia with both hands, attempt to pull the tibia forwards and note any laxity. Significant movement indicates a positive anterior drawer test – suggestive of ACL rupture.

Posterior Cruciate Ligament (PCL) – Posterior Drawer Test

- With the knee in 90° flexion and foot flat on the bed, remain sitting on their foot. Gripping their upper tibia with both hands, attempt to push the tibia posteriorly with respect to the femur and note any significant movement or laxity suggesting PCL rupture.

Medial Collateral Ligament (MCL)

- With the knee in 20° flexion, stabilise the leg with one hand. With the other hand, push the knee medially to stress the MCL. This test is performed in 20° flexion to keep the capsule and other ligaments lax to try and avoid them providing additional stability.

Lateral Collateral Ligament (LCL)

- With the knee in 20° flexion, stabilise the leg with one hand. With the other hand, push the knee laterally to stress the LCL.

Examine the opposite knee using the above steps for comparison.

For completeness, offer to examine the ipsilateral hip and ankle (as pain in one joint can often be referred from a pathology in another). Additionally, you can offer to examine the lower limbs neurologically and you may wish to assess gait.

To conclude your examination, thank the patient, wash your hands, summarise your findings to patient and examiner, and recommend further investigations if applicable.

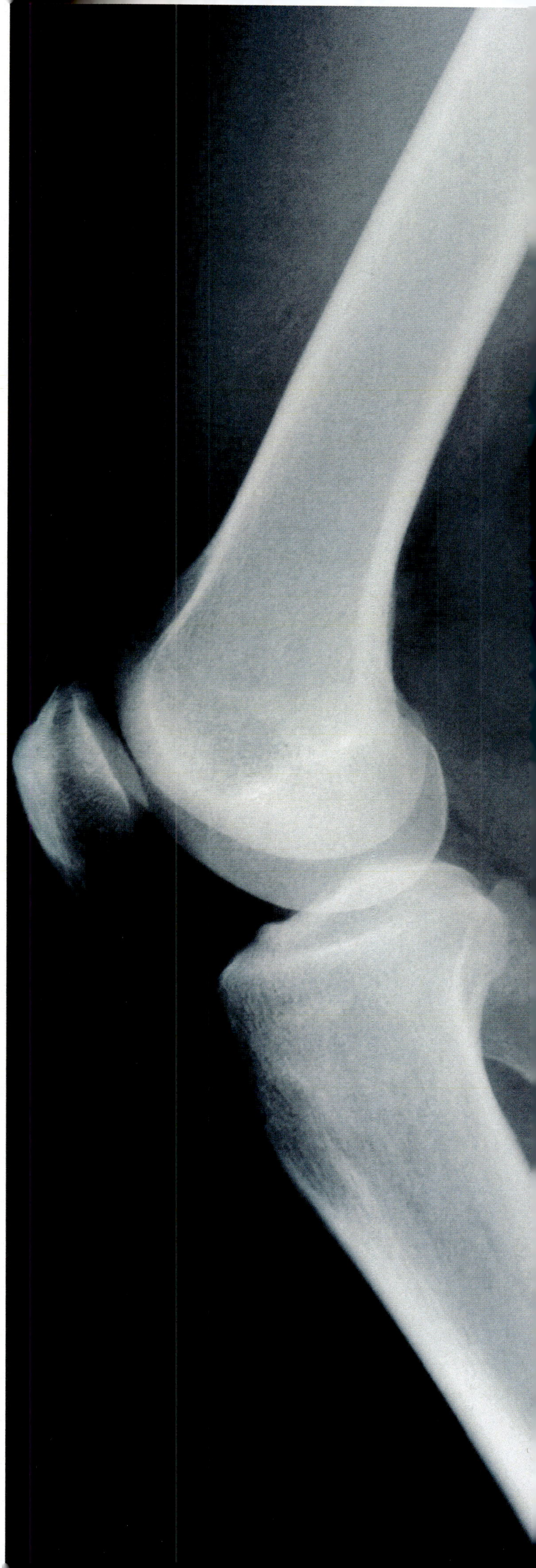

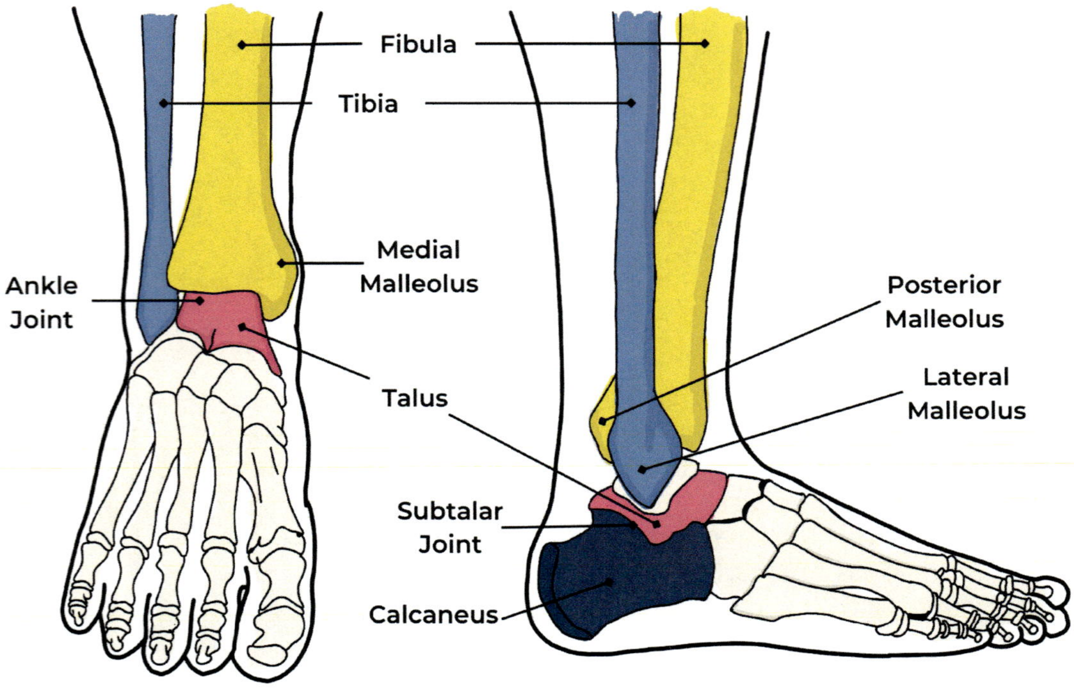

Chapter 8: Ankle & Foot Examination

Dr Katriona Hutchison BSc MBChB

The ankle and foot together are composed of 28 bones and over 30 joints. The most essential joints to be aware of for clinical examination are the 'ankle' joint and the subtalar joint. The 'ankle' joint is made from the articulation of the tibia, fibula and talus. This is a hinge joint therefore allowing plantarflexion (flexion) and dorsiflexion (extension). The subtalar joint exists between the talus and the calcaneus and is classified as a plane joint, allowing inversion and eversion of the ankle.

When examining the foot and ankle, it is important to go slowly and systematically to assess all movements.

As with all examinations, prior to examining the patient, you should introduce yourself, confirm the patient's name and date of birth, explain what the examination entails and gain patient consent.

LOOK

To be able to adequately visualise the joint, ask the patient to remove any shoes/socks and raise any trousers so the joint itself and the muscles in the lower leg can be seen. To effectively examine the feet and ankles you will need to examine the patient both when lying down and when standing.

*Tip – before assessing the patient start by looking at their footwear! Look for any signs of wear and tear which can indicate not only reasons for trauma to the foot but their gait patterns.

Supine – inspect the dorsal and plantar surfaces of the foot

- Skin Changes – inspect for rashes, scars, wounds/ulcers, calluses, nail changes
- Deformity – assess for any deformities of the joints including hallux valgus, clawing of joints
- Swelling – look for swelling over joint sites

*Tip – Always look between the toes for ulcers as these can be easily missed!

Standing – Inspect the anterior, posterior, medial and lateral surfaces of the foot/ankle joint

- Assess the arches of the feet – do they appear to be flattened or high
  - If the arch appears to be flat ask the person to stand on their tip toes to assess if the flattened arch persists
- Look for varus or valgus deformities – although not a deformity of the ankle this can give insight into issues

presenting as ankle/foot problems

- Assess for toe alignment and any deformities when standing
- Check the ankle and Calcaneal (Achilles) tendon for any swelling
- Compare calf muscles for discrepancy in size and signs of muscle wasting

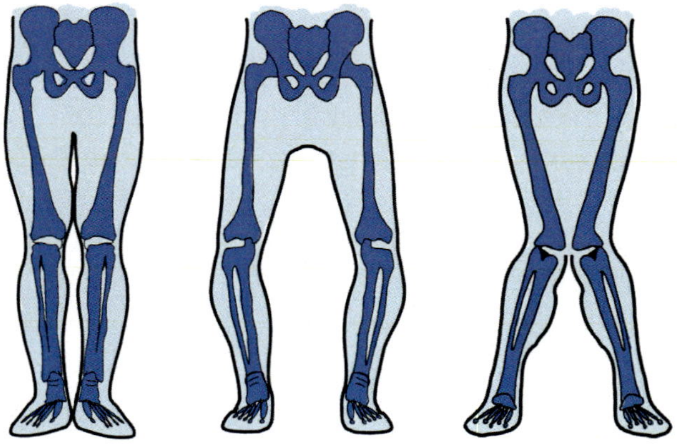

FEEL

Prior to palpation remember to check with the patient if they have any pain in their feet/ankles. Start by palpating generally across the ankle and down the foot for any changes in temperature or obvious signs of swelling. Then assess for tenderness in specific areas by palpating the following bony landmarks:

- Ankle – palpate the medial and lateral malleoli and around the anterior, posterior, medial and lateral joint lines
- Subtalar joint and midfoot – gently squeeze just below the ankle joint
- Squeeze the dorsum of the foot slowly moving distally to assess the tarsals and metatarsals.
- Squeeze the metatarsal heads where they attach to the phalanges and the interphalangeal joints individually.

*Tip – palpate the Achilles tendon to assess for any pain/thickening and the calf muscle bulk to assess for any muscle wasting.

Finally palpate posterior tibial and dorsalis pedis pulses.

MOVE

On movement of the ankle/foot joints remember to assess both passive and active movement. Assess the following movements in the supine position:

- Dorsiflexion (ankle)– pull foot/ankle back towards the body
- Plantarflexion (ankle)– push foot towards to floor as if pressing on the accelerator of a car
- Inversion – hold the ankle from the back to stabilise then use your other hand to move the heel medially.
- Eversion - hold the ankle from the back to stabilise then use your other hand to move the heel laterally.
- Midtarsal movements – hold the heel still with one hand then twist the forefoot medially and laterally with the other to assess the minor movements in the midtarsal joints.

After examining the ankle, ensure to assess dorsiflexion/plantarflexion of the big toe and ask patient to wiggle their toes to evaluate if they are flexing/extending as expected

Lastly assess function of the joints by watching the patient's gait. Look for classical heel strike, toe lift walking pattern and any variations of this. Watch to see if the patient's foot appears to be dragging or if they have a high-stepping gait (foot drop).

Common Signs on Examination

Foot Deformities:

- Hallux Valgus (Bunions) – lateral angulation of the big toe at the metatarsophalangeal joint. Can be linked to footwear such as high heels due to being tight at the metatarsophalangeal joints.
- Hallux Rigidus – swollen, stiff big toe with limited ranged of movement. Often secondary to osteoarthritis of the first metatarsophalangeal joint.
- Hammer Toe – the proximal interphalangeal joint is fixed in flexion and the distal interphalangeal joint is hyperextended
- Mallet Toe – the distal interphalangeal joint is fixed in flexion
- Claw Toe – the metatarsophalangeal joint is hyperextended and the

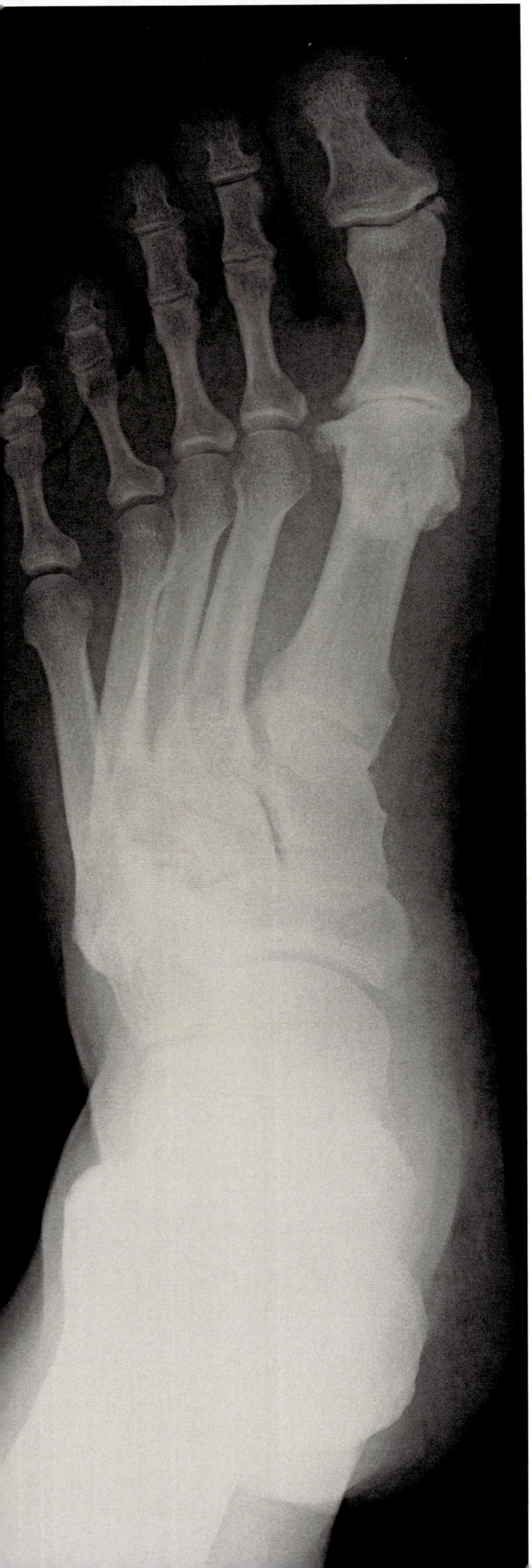

Achilles Tendonitis and Tendon Rupture

- Inflammation of the tendon sheath of the calcaneal tendon due to degeneration or overuse.
- Key Signs – pain during or following exercise, if sudden pain at back of ankle during exercise (for example when running or jumping) this could indicate tendon rupture.
- Can assess for rupture using Simmond's Test – ask patient to kneel on a chair with their feet dangling off the front of the seat. Ask the patient to relax their muscles, and then one at a time, squeeze the patient's calves. On squeezing the calf, the patient's foot should plantarflex – if this is absent then this indicates Achilles tendon rupture.

Gout

- Inflammatory arthritis secondary to deposition of urate crystals in the joints – most commonly caused by alcohol, but also linked to renal impairment, diuretics, diabetes and poor diet. Very commonly effects the 1st metatarsophalangeal joint.
- Key signs: hot, swollen, red big toe. When gout flares it is characterised by acute onset severe pain. Tophi (white crystals) can be visualised on bony prominences in some cases.

Flat Foot (Pes Planus)

- Very common, particularly in children.
- Common Signs – Flattened arch of the foot – this can be flexible, where it resolves on plantarflexion (standing on tip toes), or rigid, where the flattened arch does not resolve.

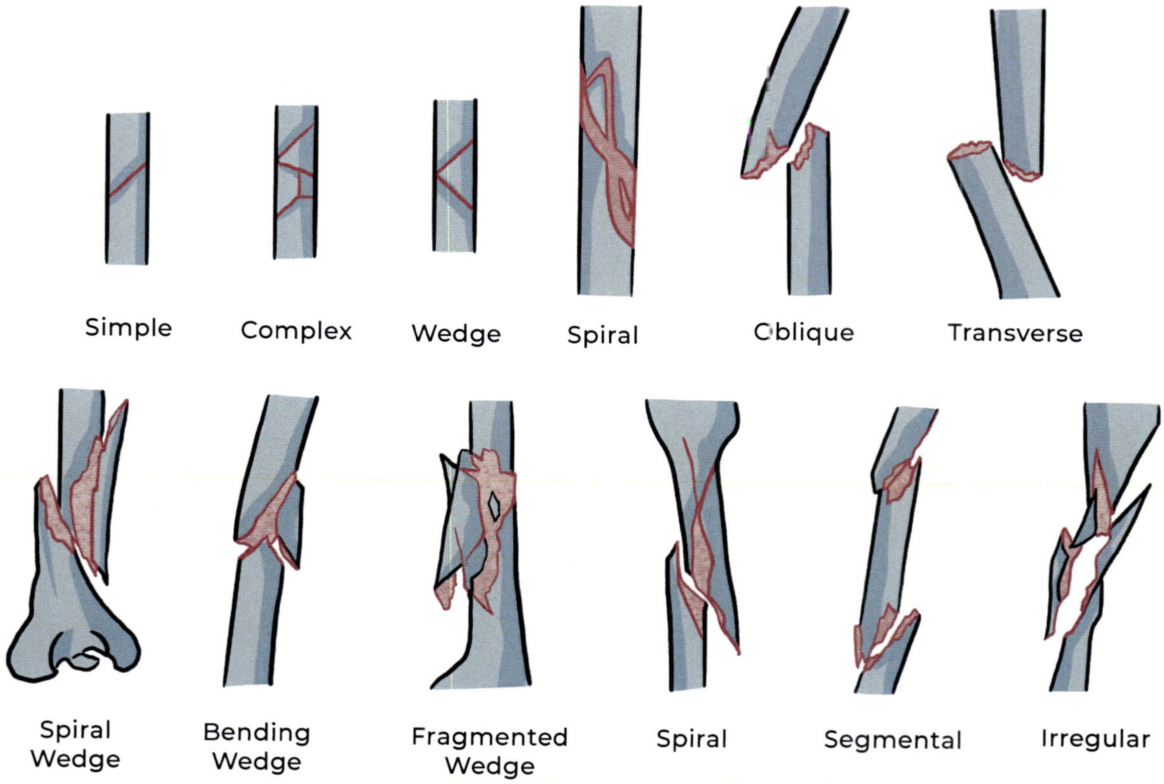

Chapter 9: Musculoskeletal Imaging & Interpretation of Common Fractures of the Limbs

Dr. Michael Carvill BMBS, BMedSci, PGDip

Approaching the Interpretation Station

Although OSCEs usually only contain one or two stations on interpretation of investigations, being able to confidently interpret any investigation will allow your other knowledge to shine through.

This chapter will focus on developing a structure for musculoskeletal radiological examination, however, many of the early tips in this chapter will also translate over to any interpretation station, be that blood results, ECGs, or other radiological investigations.

Imaging Modalities

X-Ray

Colloquially used to refer to plain film, x-rays are also used in fluoroscopy (such as seen during interventional procedures), and computed tomography (CT) scans. The varying absorption (or attenuation) of the x-ray beam by the tissues of the body, results in changes in contrast on the final image. Air will attenuate the least while fat, water, bone, and metal will attenuate to greater extents and therefore appear increasingly 'white' on the final image. The degree to which this attenuation occurs depends on the density of the structure. Tightly adjacent structures of similar density (such as soft tissues) cannot be easily distinguished on an x-ray.

Ultrasound

Ultrasound machines use a transducer which generates high-frequency sound waves. These sound waves pass through tissue and the subsequent reflections are detected and converted into images. The image is a result of calculating the time for the wave to return and the direction it returns from. Unlike an x-ray which produces an image based on attenuation through a material, the ultrasound image is based on echogenicity. A hyperechoic structure such as bone reflects the wave back and appears white, whilst decreasingly hypoechoic structures will appear dark as the wave pass through and are not reflected.

Magnetic Resonance Imaging (MRI)

MRI has particular use in the evaluation of joints – looking at the ligaments, menisci, labrum, cartilage, and capsule along with the muscles and tendons. Masses in soft tissue or bone can be assessed and staged as appropriate. Note, it is unlikely you would be asked to interpret an MRI at this stage.

Selecting the Modality for Musculoskeletal Presentations

- X-ray plain films – generally the first choice for suspected bone and joint anomalies. Remember to get two-views which include the distal and proximal joints and ask for another if you are only presented with one.
- CT – can be used in more complex fracture cases or perhaps where better evaluation of the soft tissue is required.
- Ultrasound - Used to look at tendons for damage and detect foreign bodies. Biopsies can be taken under ultrasound guidance.
- MRI - For joints the MRI can give good information regarding the structures of the joint such as the ligaments, menisci and cartilage. It also has use in soft tissue and bony mass investigations.

Approaching the X-Ray

When approaching any OSCE station it is important to have a structure. This structure of musculoskeletal X-ray interpretation will allow you to have a system to follow to ensure that you have covered all essential elements of the musculoskeletal x-ray.

Identification

- Check the patient details on the study are correct for the patient you are investigating. The name, hospital number, and date of birth should match.
- Make note of the date and ensure it is the most recent study (you can also compare to older X-rays later).
- Identify the type of imaging used (plain film, CT, US, MRI).
- Be clear on the site of the body being imaged. To help distinguish the left and right you can look out for the label on the plain film or check the name of the investigation to help guide you (although mistakes do happen, and this isn't 100% reliable).

The First Impression

- Providing that you have seen X-rays of that joint before you may already have an understanding of what normal anatomy looks like and as such, could offer a first impression before working systematically.
- After completing the identification step take a moment to look at the image. Does it look like others you have seen before? Are there any obvious abnormalities? Does it appear completely normal?
- You can then offer your first impression – for example "Upon first inspection this appears to be a normal x-ray of the hand, however, I will work through it systematically to ensure that is the case."

*Tip: you can use a similar technique for ECGs, chest X-rays, and interpretation of blood results. This first impression gives you a moment to collect your thoughts before moving to a detailed analysis.

Soft Tissue

- Better appreciated with direct clinical observation, however you can make some comments on the soft tissue from the imaging. Look for soft tissue swelling and if there is an obvious open component e.g. a fracture.

Joints

- Comment on the alignment and overall symmetry of the joint. Look at the spaces between the articular surfaces and look for evidence of osteophytes or effusions. The articular surfaces should also be examined for erosions and subchondral cysts.

Bone

- Look at the overall quality of the bone in terms of density, trabeculae, or the presence of any lesions. Trace around the cortex checking for disruption.

After your initial examination of the x-ray, look more closely at any area that does not appear normal.

- Fractures and Dislocations
  - Locate the injured bone and name it
  - What part of the bone is fractured and is it intra- or extra-articular
  - Is it simple or comminuted fracture
  - What is the direction of the line of fracture (transverse, oblique, spiral etc.)
  - Is there angulation (describe in relation of the distal segment to the proximal bone)
  - Is there translation (amount of movement between two ends of a fracture), shortening or rotation?

*Tip: when describing fractures it is tempting to stop after describing the bony injury. Remember to also comment upon soft tissue, foreign bodies, and other existing pathology.

Closing and presenting your findings

- Summarise significant findings
- Consider if any additional imaging is needed – perhaps you were only provided with a single x-ray view and therefore you should request another. If you have a fracture or dislocation, you may want to suggest a repeat x-ray following manipulation.
- Remember to compare to previous imaging where possible – this can help assess for disease progression and also work out what may be 'new' in this imaging which is relevant to the current case.

Common Upper Limb Fractures

Colles Fracture

- Distal radius fracture with dorsal angulation and displacement (a 'dinner fork' deformity)
- Views required – PA and lateral

Smith's Fracture

- Distal radius fracture with volar angulation and displacement
- Views required – PA and lateral

Humeral Shaft Fracture

- Various patterns of injury – it is important to be able to distinguish the various types of humeral fractures on the image on the begining of this chapter.
- Views required – AP and lateral

Colles Fracture

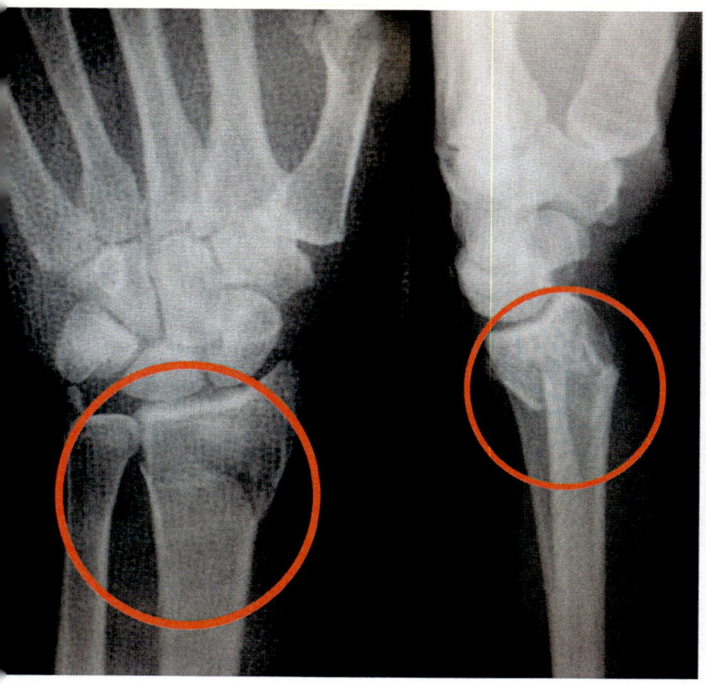

Smith's Fracture

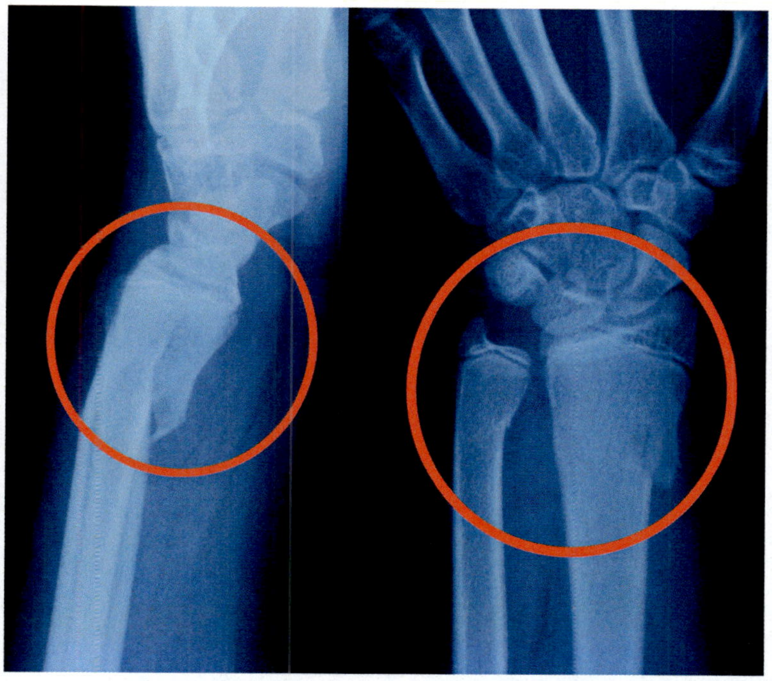

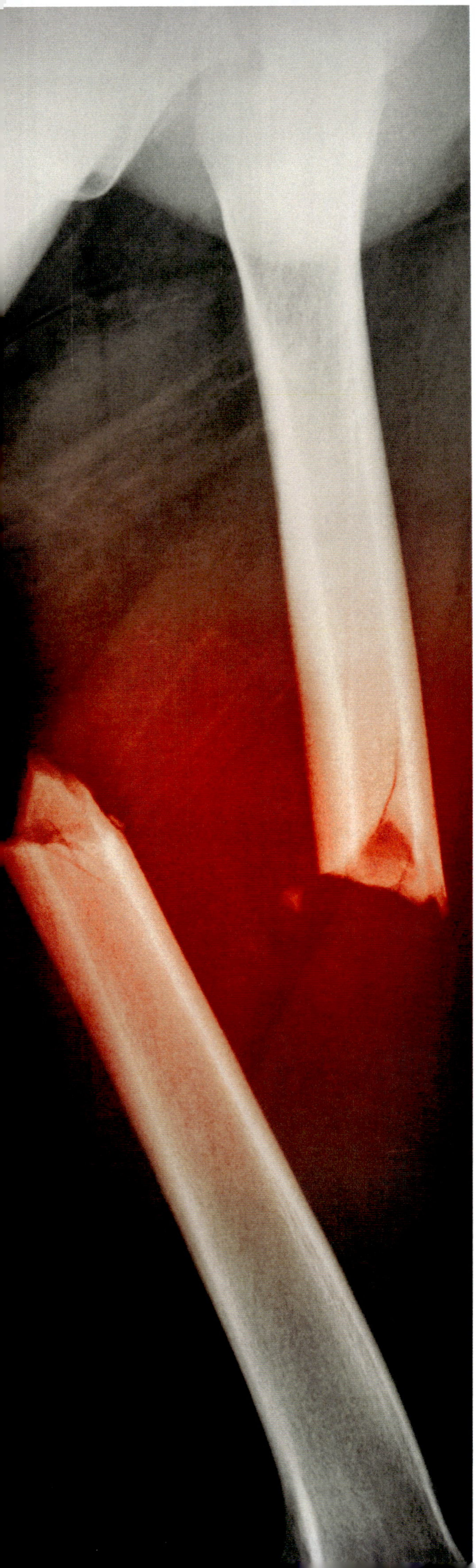

Common Lower Limb Fractures

Femoral Shaft Fracture

- Various patterns of injury – as with humeral fractures take note of the various types of femoral fractures in the image below.
- Views required – AP and lateral of the femur, AP and lateral of the hip, AP and lateral of the knee

Tibial Shaft Fracture

- Various patterns of injury
- Views required – AP and lateral of the tibia, AP, lateral and oblique of the knee, AP, lateral and oblique of the ankle

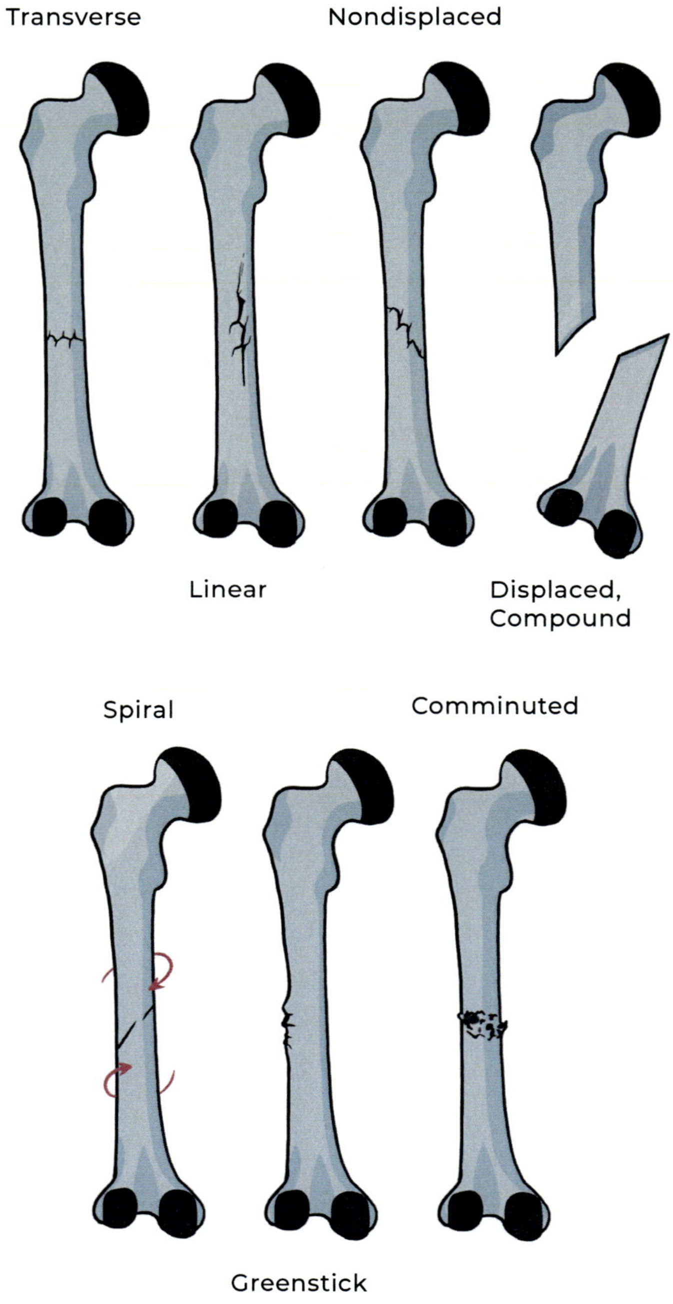

Made in the USA
Las Vegas, NV
09 January 2026

38862543R00024